The Cancer in the American Healthcare System

POST OBAMACARE EDITION

How Washington Controls And Destroys Our Health Care

Dr. Deane Waldman, MD MBA

Strategic Book Publishing and Rights Co.

ISBN: 978-1-68181-381-3 softcover

Library of Congress Control Number: 2015950588

Part of the proceeds from this book will be contributed to the Wounded Veterans Initiative developed by Canine Companions for Independence®.

Cover Design: Len Williams, www.designstrategies.com

Interior Layout: & Formatting: Ronda Taylor, www.taylorbydesign.com

Strategic Book Publishing & Rights Co., LLC
USA | Singapore
www.sbpra.com

Praise for *The Cancer In Healthcare* [2012]

The Cancer In Healthcare is an "easy, entertaining read ... it will make the Bad Guys squirm.... Dr. Waldman's style is lively and lucid, and the book is packed with facts. It is not just another boring recital of platitudes.... His real life examples leave no doubt as to how absurd and sick the system is.... Read it and weep, laugh, or both."

Jane Orient MD, 4 out of 5 stars

"I learned so much from reading this book. Now I'm even more terrified about our state of affairs than I ever was before.... This book ... completely opened my mind to the causes of our problems. It is easy to read and very informative. I highly recommend that you read it."

S. Curley, 5 out of 5 stars

"Although timely for a number of reasons, perhaps the most relevant comments are reserved for the Affordable Care Act ... Waldman does a good job of showing how the rules and regulations of this act will lead to even higher healthcare costs and the rationed treatment ... it's a quick, easy, and lively read, one full of examples."

Doug Erlandson, Amazon Top 500 Reviewer, 5 out of 5 stars

"Easy to understand. A fast fun read that will help you get a better understanding of the issues with U.S. healthcare ... easy for anyone reading it to understand, but does not lack real fact-based academic rigor.

S. Power, Amazon Top 500 Reviewer, 5 out of 5 stars

"I recommend this book for anyone who wants to better understand why health care is failing and be inspired to change our course ... My favorite part of the book is the last chapter, which encourages individual empowerment ... If we continue to allow the government to 'spend' our way out of trouble, we will simply continue to grow the cancer."

Leah Oviedo, 4 out of 5 stars

"This book provides a startling series of examples of just how much patient care has been replaced by red tape ... a great eye opening read."

"Dr. Waldman has hit the nail squarely on the head. Bureaucratic greed has destroyed the finest health care system the world has ever known."

Preface to This "Post Obamacare" Edition

In 2012, when the Supreme Court upheld Obamacare, I gave up practicing medicine. I didn't want to quit as I loved caring for small children. However, my personal moral code prevented me from participating in a federal fiction, especially one that would hurt my patients.

Tort law very clearly states that only a licensed physician can practice medicine. Yet a different law, the Affordable Care Act, gives a newly created arm of the federal government called the Independent Payment Advisory Board, the power to do just that—to practice medicine. This agency, which is composed of political appointees and meets in secret, has the power to over-rule my medical recommendations. They can tell me what I am not allowed to do medically, even though what I propose could save a patient. I refuse to accept responsibility for the welfare of a patient when a government committee is making all the medical decisions.

I decided to combine my experience being a doctor with my business knowledge and figure out what was really wrong with the American healthcare system. What is going on—what is the root cause of healthcare's fall from grace? Was Obamacare making things better or worse? Most important, what would it take for the U.S. to have a system that improved the health of all Americans and didn't drive our nation into bankruptcy?

This book answers those questions. I call it the Post Obamacare Edition for two reasons. First, since the ACA was implemented in 2014, we have *evidence* of its effect. We can now assess Obamacare based not on predictions or promises but on hard facts.

In the last chapter, I ask (and answer) what if Obamacare were repealed? What if we lived in a "Post Obamacare" world? What should we do with healthcare? It turns out to be rather simple, as all good things are.

We can take back control of our health care and restore our once-great healthcare system at the same time. The cure is simple. It is neither quick nor easy.

Dr. Deane Waldman, July 4, 2015

Dedication

Over my thirty-seven years as a pediatric cardiologist, I had the privilege of caring for thousands of children with heart problems. Every morning when I got up, I smiled at the day ahead. I got to *play* with children and people even paid me to do it!

All of my former patients are now old enough to read. I dedicate this book to them.

My patients were the recipients of health care in a system that committed itself to their welfare as its highest priority, above all other things like budget constraints, government rules, insurance regulations, or political advantage. THAT system is fading. It has an out of control cancer.

I hope my patients, and patients everywhere (which means everyone), will read this book, discard the *wisdom* that says healthcare can't be fixed, and like a good doctor, do "whatever it takes" to restore our system for medical care to good health and optimal function.

Contents

and experienced pediatric cardiologist, not to some bureaucrat whom they had never met.

Lily's family paid their hard-earned money to the insurance company. Didn't the company care at all about Lily?

Here's another thing that threw me. Lily's operation cost over a quarter of a million dollars. Why was insurance jeopardizing an investment of hundreds of thousand dollars to save a couple hundred bucks? Worse, if Lily had taken the medications that her insurance company "approved," she would've quickly ended up in the Intensive Care Unit, which would have cost the insurance company far more than the measly $563 a month in medications.

That was my first indication that something was seriously wrong with the system, a system that (I thought) was there to help me take care of patients. It wasn't just a few bad apples. It was the system!

Lily's scenario is now so commonplace that we take it for granted. We accept the unacceptable. Why? Because instead of expecting doctors and nurses to care for our health (what we used to think of as *health care*—two words), we have resigned ourselves to being victimized by the system called *healthcare* (one word).

Health care (two words) = **services and products**
Healthcare (one word) = a **system** to provide those services and goods

---

The conversion of health care from a mom-and-pop operation to a massive, complex industrial system was finished by the 1980s. I saw this directly with my mother-in-law. Her name was Pearl, and it was a perfect name for her. She was a real gem. I had a relationship with her most sons-in-law can only envy. In her seventies, Pearl began to develop arthritis in her hips. She went to see the doctor and afterward reported her experience.

She told me "they" prescribed some medications and an exercise program. Surgery might be necessary in the future but hopefully, she could avoid it. When I asked her the name of her doctor, she replied, "Northwestern." She was referring to a very large, high quality health system in Chicago called Northwestern Memorial Hospitals. I knew it well as I trained there after medical school.

I repeated my question, "Northwestern, well of course, but who is your doctor?"

To which my mother-in-law answered (again), "Northwestern. I never got a doctor's name. I am not sure even they know *my* name. They never used it."

Once upon a time, the United States of America had health care (two words). This involved a close personal relationship between a patient and a doctor. When we still had health care, your doctor still cared about you, as a person.

Say that you developed a symptom such as chest pain or a sign like a rash. You would immediately pick up the phone and call your doctor's office, a number you knew well. This is the conversation you were likely to have. (Note when your call was picked up, you got a human, not an automatic message with a flat, artificial computer voice.)

Office: Dr. So-and-So's office. This is Ruth. How may we help you?

You: Ruth, this is Mrs. Smith. I am calling …

Ruth (interrupting): Gladys, good to hear your voice. How is everyone in the family, especially that handsome husband of yours? Is everything okay? Do you have a problem?

You: I am not sure. I think I might need to see Dr. Jones.

Ruth: Well, of course. If you are concerned, you should talk with him.

You: I know how busy he is. Any chance for an appointment, maybe next week?

Ruth: A week?! Don't be silly. If you are concerned, we will get you in right away. I can add you after today's last patient. Come in around 7:00 p.m. Will that work?

You: Really, you don't have to make him stay late.

Ruth: If you are concerned, then he is concerned. He won't be able to relax until he makes sure there is nothing serious going on. Come in and we will take care of you.

You: Thank you so much. I cannot tell you how relieved I am.

---

you cannot simply cut out the liver or destroy all the blood cells. The patient cannot survive without a liver or without blood cells.

Cancer cells are strong, tough, and very greedy. Sometimes the treatment can kill the patient. Chemotherapy and radiation kills both healthy as well as cancerous cells. The idea is to kill all the cancer cells but not so many healthy ones that the patient dies. This is a tricky balancing act. Once the cancer is gone, the remaining healthy cells can grow and eventually restore the patient to good health.

Just as a human cannot survive without a liver, so the government cannot function without a bureaucracy. Curing the cancer in bureaucracy requires restoring control of the bureaucracy to the people, taking it away from the cancer.

Treating any cancer successfully, in a human or in a bureaucracy, requires a medical commitment to do "whatever it takes," not a political approach of negotiation and compromise. Your doctor doesn't negotiate with a malignant tumor agreeing to take out only part of it. There is no compromise with leukemia, not if you want to end up with a healthy patient.

Over the years, you and I have seen various "fixes" for our healthcare system, or you could call them "treatments" for sick patient healthcare. The Affordable Care Act (ACA), what we have come to call Obamacare, is just the latest in a long line.[1]

We all hoped that Obamacare was going to fix the sick system. As an experienced doctor, I wasn't optimistic, and unfortunately, my worst fears were well founded.

- Insurance premiums are far higher than they were before ACA.
- Doctors and other health-care professionals are leaving the profession in droves.
- People are no longer able to use their family doctor.
- Veterans cannot get the care they need to stay alive.
- And, we are spending more than ever!

Despite the best of intentions, Washington's "fixes" have actually *fueled the cancer's growth.*

Unless we face up to the root cause of our failing healthcare system, we're not going to be able to fix it. Only when we learn what is really encouraging the uncontrolled greed and unrestrained power will we be able to reclaim that which belongs to us: our health, our wellbeing, and our ability to "live long and prosper" —Mr. Spock's customary salutation on science fiction series *Star Trek*.[2]

Until we accept that cancer is sucking the life out of the American healthcare system, our dreams will keep turning into nightmares.

ONE

Dreams of Healthcare

What do you dream about? Living in a grand house? Having a successful career? We often dream about things we want such as having a great car or taking a luxury vacation. We sometimes dream about being acknowledged for the hard work we've done, like winning a prestigious award or getting a substantial raise. Some of you might even dream about making it big on stage or screen.

Even though you might not be aware of it, you also dream about having good health or being healthy. After all, you cannot enjoy that convertible BMW if you are unable to drive it. It is hard for you to accept your Nobel Prize from a hospital bed. You can't be a star if you're too sick to work all the hours it takes to be a success—from making the movies to constantly looking your best.

In other words, everyone's dreams of success presume that we are healthy and that we live a long time.

To say that the passage of Obamacare was and still is contentious is an understatement. But putting politics aside for a moment, let's look at why some kind of reform was absolutely necessary. Prior to Barack Obama taking office with his promise of healthcare reform, our healthcare system wasn't fulfilling our dreams. It was the stuff of nightmares.

We live in the richest and most powerful nation on earth. By every measure, we have the most productive people and the highest standard of living. We should have the best health care on earth. We should expect the following:

- A healthcare industry that remembers that people come first, ahead of money.
- Getting whatever medical care we need, when we need it.
- The ability to go to any doctor we want to when we need to.

We all assume that our health care provider will restore our health when we are sick and fix any long-standing problems. Whatever our medical concerns, our doctor can and should solve them.

I think many of us still dream about having a Marcus Welby-type doctor. *Marcus Welby, MD* was a very popular TV show that aired from 1969 to 1976. It starred Robert Young, James Brolin, and Elena Verdugo. The title character was a general practitioner who had time for everyone: patients, friends, and neighbors alike. He always had the right answer for whatever problem(s) you had. The name "Marcus Welby" became synonymous with the perfect physician. Unfortunately, HMOs cured us of that ideal thirty years ago. However, we still believe that our doctors, nurses, and other healthcare professionals will have our best interests at heart. (And we always hope, with a little hand wringing, that our healthcare expenses won't cause us heart failure).

There are those who have come to expect the government to take care of us, particularly those who are less fortunate. None of us wants to hear about anyone being denied life-saving care simply because they are poor. But when we get sick, we have one goal—to get better—and we expect our doctors, nurses, hospitals, and our insurance companies to have that same goal.

Even though we all agree that our health is our own responsibility, health-care providers are responsible for the quality of care that we get. When they harm you, they should be punished—and so sometimes we may have dreams of vengeance, or at least justice, depending on how you want to phrase it.

Bottom line: all of us know what we really want from healthcare (the system)—good health care (two words) from someone who cares about our health before all else. Everyone everywhere wants the exact same thing. I do mean everyone and everywhere. We want to survive, not just barely but with abundance. As I said in the introduction, we all want to "live long and prosper." (Incidentally, Leonard Nimoy, who played Spock, says that he got the saying from ancient Hebrew texts.)

"Live long" means being alive into our eighties, nineties, or beyond. It wasn't that long ago that reaching a hundred years of age produced a newspaper article. Now, greeting card companies sell numerous varieties of cards that celebrate a hundredth birthday.

"Prosper" means to have an abundance of both money as well as health. What good is having a big bank account without the ability to enjoy it?

The question is this: if the healthcare system is afflicted to its core with cancer, is it even possible to "live long and prosper?"

Do Providers Dream?

Because I am a doctor, I feel I must address both sides of the health-care equation: patients *and* providers. Even though we doctors are sometimes made out to be the patient's enemy, providers' dreams are very much the same as yours.

On an individual level, we dream of *having* the same things that you do: a healthy, loving family, a nice home, comfortable living, and a long time to enjoy these things. At some point in our lives, every provider becomes a patient.

Providers—your doctors, nurses, and allied health personnel—have dreams of both having and *doing*. With major medical advances happening, sometimes routinely, we want to do better for our patients now than we did in the past because we *can*.

I vividly recall my Uncle Martyn. He was a physician, just like his dad, my grandfather. He was a thoracic surgeon, or what they called in the 1970 satire movie *M*A*S*H*, a "chest-cutter." When I was a young boy, I remember him telling me that he dreamed of replacing a heart that did not work with a new one, like changing worn out tires on your car. That was his impossible dream fifty years ago. Today, it is routine—an everyday reality.

As providers, we dream about advances in medicine and medical technology that can help our patients live longer lives and be more prosperous.

As a physician, I also dream about doing better for my patients, one in particular. I might have had some patients who were cuter than Matt (maybe, but I doubt it). I treated thousands of cute babies and adorable children. Matt still is my favorite patient after forty-one years of practice because he was special. He was unique.

I still dream that he could have lived.

Matt was born in 1979 with a very abnormal heart. Where you and I have four valves, two pumping chambers, and two "great arteries," Matt had two valves, one pump, and one artery. Even as a baby, he was Matt, not some nickname or even Mattie. When Matt was nine months old, his mother started calling him her "little old man."

We did a number of procedures and gave him medications to help him survive, even grow, but we could not fix his heart completely. No one knew how.

I studied, tested, and tested again. Eventually, I invented a new operation, just for Matt. This operation fixed his heart problem. It separated the red (oxygenated) blood from the blue blood (without oxygen) and made him dramatically better. He went home four days after an operation that had never been done before, pink (not blue) for the first time in his short life.

Unfortunately, the operation only worked for five more years. It became clear Matt was dying. His was born in May 1979. In January 1988, he told his mother he "wasn't going to make it, so could they have his ninth birthday party in February?"

Of course, she said yes. We all had a wonderful time. At his party, Matt announced to all that when he died, he was going to come back as a blue-eyed elephant. In private, he told me that he had a present for me, but he would "give it to me later." He did not say when.

Matt died in April, one month before his ninth birthday. He had given his pastor specific instructions about the funeral. (I told you he had a wise old head.) He wanted only his mother and Dr. Deane to speak, and I had to go second. When I got up to the podium, I saw that he had instructed his mother to put a little charm of a tricycle there as my present. Matt knew of my love of bicycling. The charm remains in front of me today, on my bookshelves next to my desk.

I still dream that I knew then what I know now. At the time of Matt's surgery, neither we nor anyone else on earth knew it is necessary to make blood coming out of the liver go directly to the lungs. Without that small but critical flow pattern, the lungs are gradually damaged. What ultimately caused Matt's death was a big hole in the world's medical knowledge base. If we had known to add the liver flow adjustment to his procedure, Matt could be alive today.

Believe it or not, several months after Matt died, the Wild Animal Park in San Diego (where Matt's family lived) announced in the newspaper that one of their elephants was pregnant. I went with Matt's mother to talk with the animal keepers, and we told them Matt's prediction. When the baby elephant was born, we went to look, but his eyes were brown. They named him Matt anyway.

There are many people who have lived because we have dreamed of ways to fix their health problem. There are many more who have died because we didn't have the answers that we needed for them.

Hopefully, you have good health and did not have to take out a second mortgage to pay your medical bills. Hopefully, you got your mammogram on time, and they got the lump out before it became stage IV cancer. But what's becoming more and more the case is that your dreams are being thwarted because, as we know all too well, there is something desperately wrong with our healthcare system.

In fact, despite spectacular medical advances over the past century, the healthcare system has become the opposite of what we dream. Being a doctor has become a living nightmare, one that seems to be getting worse, not better.

TWO

A Waking Nightmare

Here in the United States, when we are sick, we expect our doctors, nurses, and hospitals to be there to help us, and that insurance will pay for the care we need. Unfortunately, there are too many times when our doctors, nurses, hospitals, and insurance companies fail us. You already know the story of Lily—the sweet baby that had the heart transplant but the insurance company wouldn't approve her medication until I strong-armed them to do what was right.

Reality is what we experience—what we "get." Dreams are what we wish to get. Nightmares are increasingly what we *do* get.

I hear stories all the time of healthcare nightmares, ranging from little things like a nurse accidentally putting pain meds just out of a patient's reach to horrendous nightmares like Lily's.

Even though I am a doctor, I have also been a patient. As a patient, I was not immune from having a doctor turn my healthcare dreams into nightmares. I like to ride my bicycle hard and to race when I can. That requires intense training, which I was doing early one morning when a rabbit literally ran into my front wheel. With the poor animal trapped in the spokes, the bike stopped instantly. I, of course, did not. So over the handlebars I went, breaking my fall with my hands and thereby injuring my wrist.

In the ER, even I (a cardiologist) could see the broken bones. The Chief of Orthopedic Surgery came in, examined me, and reviewed the

X-rays. He said I needed immediate surgery if I wanted to use my wrist for the delicate procedures that I do. Of course I instantly agreed to have the operation. The surgeon said he had done thousands of these, and I should make a complete recovery. In other words, he tacitly assured me that my dream of a perfect result from health care would come to pass.

The surgery went fine. Afterward, they splinted my wrist. It needed time for the swelling to go down. Ten days later, a cast was applied. I felt fine, fine enough to do some bicycle training on my stationary trainer in my garage, putting no weight on the casted wrist.

A week later, I was in Chicago, testifying in a medical malpractice case when I became deathly ill. At 4:00 a.m., I found myself in the same hospital where I had trained thirty years before. The infection was so severe that I was immediately put in the ICU and given three different intravenous antibiotics a total of nine times a day along with painkillers that kept me asleep. Due to the great care I received, I eventually recovered nearly full function. Three months later, I was again doing procedures on babies' hearts.

I suspect that the infection started when I did that indoor training and sweated under the cast. The surgeon who operated (he was the Chief of Orthopedic Surgery) *never* told me that, after this type of surgery, there was a 10 percent incidence of infection. That is one out of every ten patients!

I guess he just thought everyone knew this—either that or he assumed I knew because I was a doctor myself. Why he would believe a children's heart specialist would know the complications after bone surgery is still a mystery to me, as both patient and physician, and the consequences of that reverberate far beyond just my own injury and what it could have done to my career. It points to one of the nightmares people constantly run up against when they have contact with the healthcare system—even with the best intentions, sometimes the outcomes aren't what we want. They turn dreams into nightmares.

My good friend Dr. T. is a case in point. He was a pediatric cardiologist in another state. Like me, he did heart catheterizations in small babies. This procedure involves putting small, flexible plastic tubes called catheters in a vein of the baby's leg, advancing them up into the heart and moving them around inside that tiny heart, either for diagnosis or to actually fix things. When you are talking about a moving structure—a baby's heart is about the size of a strawberry—the physician needs great eye-hand coordination and very fine manual dexterity.

My friend was a nationally known expert in catheterization. Interestingly, while I had only known Dr. T for about twenty years, I briefly dated his older sister in my youth.

Anyway, Dr. T had what we used to call a wry neck. He had to hold his head off to one side in order to minimize the pain in his neck and shoulders that he suffered most of the time. After consulting with various doctors, my colleague-friend had an operation on his cervical spine, the spinal cord in his neck.

As a result of the surgery, the nerves going to his arms no longer transmitted impulses. Dr. T immediately lost use of both of his hands. (This gave a whole new meaning to his relationship with his wife. Just think about, ahem, bathroom activities.)

Over the next two years, Dr. T gradually recovered about 50 percent use of one hand and 70 percent of the other. He never did a catheterization again.

These stories are not rare, isolated events. They are everyday occurrences that illustrate how our dreams can quickly turn to nightmares, even within a system that is supposedly the best in the world.

The Nightmare of the Queue

In a perfect world, our health care needs are taken care of as soon as they arise. Even though we've all had bad experiences, we still like to believe that we don't need to worry about whether our insurance will cover our care or whether we will have a doctor there ready to take care of us when we need help.

We have all heard the horror stories that creep across our border from Canada as well as from across the Atlantic (England and Europe) about how people have to wait a long time to get the help they need—how they're put in a queue or a line and made to wait their turn. We've been told we don't have to worry about all that here.

A Canadian woman I know told how she had an abnormal pap smear but couldn't have the proper procedure done for months (I don't remember if it was nine months or thirteen) because there wasn't a doctor available. She considered herself lucky that the problem didn't turn into full-blown cervical cancer.

Then there was the sixty-nine year old sheep farmer in England, still working hard, who needed his appendix out. After waiting a *year*, and after getting parliament and his doctors involved, his local hospital finally agreed to do the operation. Appendix surgeries are routine. If a bad appendix bursts, it becomes life threatening.

Even though stories like these disturb us, most Americans believe these things will never happen here in the United States.

Unfortunately it does happen here, even among people who pay their insurance premiums and have done so for the past fifty years! A friend of mine recently told me about her seventy-eight-year old mother who had a prolapsed uterus.

(Men might wish to skip over this story. It could steal the romance out of your fantasies about women.)

A fairly common medical problem in older women is a gradual weakening in the walls that support the uterus so that it is no longer contained within the body. The uterus then falls into the vagina. This carries a risk of serious infection and may make urination difficult-to-impossible.

The seventy-eight-year old woman went to her doctor who correctly diagnosed the problem and recommended surgery as soon as possible. This doctor discussed with the patient the procedures including risks and benefits as well as alternative options and cost. The patient agreed to the surgery.

When the woman tried to schedule the procedure, she came face to face with an insurance bureaucracy that used the infamous "Three D" strategy—delay, defer, and deny. So this older (being her age myself, I avoid the word "elderly") woman who enjoys excellent health otherwise and leads a very active life, had to insert a device every day into her vagina. She could have left it in but it was very uncomfortable. It was a constant trade off—the discomfort of the device or the discomfort of not being able to empty her bladder. Reinserting the device was not easy, even though this woman was a trained OB-GYN nurse and knew what she was doing. She told my friend that she worried at one point that if she were eventually denied surgery, because of her age, she wouldn't be able to continue reinserting the device.

There was another very dangerous problem lurking. Every time she removed the device and reinserted it, despite the cleansing process, her risk of infection increased. She could have suffered a serious urinary tract infection that would have put her in the hospital and could have cost more than the surgery!

Did her insurance company care? Apparently not! They used every administrative tactic imaginable to avoid paying hefty sums to the hospital and the doctor. It took eight months before she had the corrective surgery.

I am pleased to report that she is now fine. However, she endured months of unnecessary discomfort and the ongoing risk of infection before insurance relented.

The Nightmare of the Underinsured

The increasing costs we pay for healthcare—through the higher insurance premiums we're all experiencing, plus the higher taxes we're all now having to pay—have become everyone's nightmare: patients, providers, and payers.

It hurts most when it is our children who are affected, like the daughter of my friend Bill.

I knew Bill two different ways. I met him first while bicycle racing on a track, called a velodrome. He was stronger than I was. Fortunately, I was in a younger age category so I did not have to race against him. Bill was also the service manager at the car dealership where I had bought and then serviced my car.

Between Bill's job and his wife's work, together they made close to $100,000 per year, putting them in the top 15 percent of wage earners in the country. Of course they had good insurance through the car dealership. When their teenage daughter was diagnosed with leukemia, they never gave a thought to the money. They just wanted to make sure their daughter stayed alive.

Their fourteen-year old had a somewhat unusual form of leukemia but still had a good chance for permanent remission. (Many cancer specialists say you cannot "cure" leukemia. You can only achieve a permanent remission.)

After seven months of chemotherapy and nine, mostly brief, hospital admissions, their daughter was free of cancer cells. I am pleased to say she has remained healthy ever since. Bill was, however, shocked to receive the bill for her care: $184, 915. The bill itself wasn't the big surprise—he knew the care was going to be expensive. The shock was how much he had to pay. The insurance company paid $110,949. This left an outstanding balance of $73,966 to be paid out of pocket.

What would you do faced with that "Bill for Payment, due in thirty days"?

Bill sat down with the hospital and arranged a payment schedule that wouldn't force him to declare bankruptcy. He paid monthly installments and continued doing so for eight years. Bill no longer raced with us. He could not afford racing tires or even entry fees. Worse, a crash was unthinkable. It might prevent him from working and thereby render it impossible to continue making his payments to the hospital.

Bill got his "dream" result *medically* but then he had to live with a *financial* nightmare.

Until the housing crash of 2008-2009, medical bills were the most common reason that Americans had to declare bankruptcy. At present, they may "only" be number two, but the specter of astronomical medical bills haunts all of us. The scary fact is, the majority of those who had to declare bankruptcy had health insurance but could not afford to pay the bills insurance did not cover.

These people are called the "underinsured." Those are individuals who have health insurance, often very strong policies, but are still at risk for subsequent medical bills—co-payments, goods and services that are not covered, or caps on payments—that they cannot pay. At least thirty million Americans are classified as underinsured.

So the hard fact is, between fifty million uninsured and thirty million underinsured, one third of the entire U.S. workforce is living the waking nightmare of healthcare—not having the means to pay for the care they need.

Provider Nightmares

Health-care providers experience nightmares too. On a personal level, I have long wished that we could grow a new heart for a person, right from his or her own cells. I dream this because I've experienced the heartbreak of losing a patient when the body rejects a transplanted heart. I cannot stop it, and worse, what if medicine will find the cure right after the next patient dies—like my favorite, Matt? If medicine learns how to grow a new heart from existing cells, then suddenly, all the problems of transplanting someone else's heart into you—the fear of rejection, complications from the medicines, and danger of infection—would simply disappear.

Providers constantly dream about what we wish we could do for and with our patients. We would love to have the luxury of time—time to talk with you and form a close personal connection with you. We all dream of having whatever resources we need to provide the best possible care and the knowledge to cure you, not just make you feel better.

However, practicing medicine has become a continuous nightmare for every doctor and nurse. Providers keep asking themselves why the "system" that is supposed to help us care for you has made it increasingly impossible to do that. *It makes no sense.*

Most providers take the time to ensure that we're continually trained on the latest medicine and the most effective procedures that will keep our patients healthy. Meanwhile, insurance companies try to prevent us from providing any care that is expensive.

Pharmaceutical companies charge outrageous prices for many of the common drugs patients need. A portion of those charges is profit. A large chunk goes for lobbying and part will pay the costs for more specialized drugs that can make miracles happen but insurance companies won't pay for them. The result is that many miracles are put beyond the financial reach of patients. When you add in all the government regulations—most of which simply waste providers' time—it's a wonder any care is given at all. And wait until you see, later in this book, what ACA does.

I never learned to accept it when some non-physician bureaucrat would try to tell me that I wasn't allowed to treat a patient the best way I knew how. I hated it when a hospital tried to stop me from admitting a patient because there was no identifiable payment source. Providers are not interested in escape clauses, lawyerly phrases, or weasel words.

Personally, I don't give a da*n about the patient's finances. The patient is sick and needs care, *now.* Since I know what to do, I feel, like every other provider, ethically bound to provide that care. Period. I can't count how many times I had to buck the system to help someone who couldn't pay, or who was denied the treatments I prescribed, just because the insurance company said so. If I hadn't retired, I would be feeling the effects of ACA. I would be even more hampered in my efforts to cure you because, as I learned long ago, the government thinks it must create regulations to protect *you* from *me*, your doctor.

You probably know that more and more doctors are quitting clinical practice, but do you know why? Most are giving up because they can't practice medicine at the level of quality the patients expect to receive and that we doctors want to deliver.

The thing that is driving us out of the noble work we have spent years of our lives learning how to do is clear. In this new age of greedy insurance companies, coupled with too much government regulation, as a patient you are no longer able to get what you want, what you need, and what you should expect from your healthcare system.

Caring for others, especially for sick people, should give doctors and nurses the greatest professional as well as personal satisfaction. But that dream, too, has become a nightmare.

National Nightmares

The United States of America was founded by a courageous people. We banded together to declare our freedom from tyranny. It was a powerful experiment, one that has survived over two hundred years because each succeeding generation has perpetuated that dream of freedom.

We want our great nation to remain a place for optimists, where you see opportunities not roadblocks, where you know that your children will have a better life than you do.

Alexis de Tocqueville, the famous French nineteenth-century social and political thinker, wrote in his *Democracy in America* that he saw a new nation with unbounded potential. He observed a culture that saw only limitless opportunities, and wrote, "When the privileges and disqualifications of class have been abolished, … the idea of progress comes naturally into every man's mind; the desire and ability to rise swells in every heart at once."[1]

As Americans, we want to thrive, not merely survive. We see infinite possibilities. We are certain we can improve our competitive position on the global stage.

It is almost unthinkable to us that our country might have to declare bankruptcy and become non-competitive in the global economy. Heaven forbid we lose our dominance as the world's most powerful nation. But these impossibilities are becoming not only possible but maybe even probable! We are living a waking nightmare that we can't fix, caused by a cancer that is fueled by greed and a hunger for power.

One of the most obvious indications that something is out of control is this: in 2014, we spent much more per person *per capita* than any other nation in the world. Check out the following table. Notice that we spent fifty percent more than the country in second place (Switzerland) and double what Germany, Canada, and France each spend on their people. When you compare spending on healthcare by percent of GDP, no one even comes close.

All these frightening numbers are *before* the huge costs of ACA kicked in.

Spending on Healthcare by Country		
Country	**Annual USD ($) per capita (2014)**	**% GDP (2013)**
United States	8745	17.1
Switzerland	6080	11.5
Germany	4811	11.3
Canada	4602	10.9
France	4288	11.7
Australia	3997	9.0
Japan	3649	10.3
United Kingdom	3289	9.1

You now ask the key question: what does the U.S. get by spending close to nine thousand dollars a year for each and every person in our country? Answer: we certainly don't get a fraction of the kind of service that amount of money should buy.

We rank number forty in longevity out of 135 nations—that means Americans don't live as long as the people in thirty-nine other nations. Japan is number one in longevity of its people, and they spend less than half of what we do on healthcare.

We are number thirty-four in the world in infant mortality—a statistic that should disturb everyone. We also have the dubious honor of being ranked number eighty-one in hospital beds per one-thousand people, meaning eighty countries have more hospital beds than the U.S. does despite spending less, sometimes far less, than what we spend on our healthcare.

The U.S. is fifty-second in how many doctors we have per capita (2.3/1000 people). We do, however, have more lawyers (3.7/1,000) than any other country in the world. We are also number one in something we would rather not be: obesity: 30.6 percent of our population is classified as obese. The next closest nation is Mexico at 24 percent.

All these statistics boil down to this: we're spending the most dollars but not getting the most value for those dollars, not by a very long shot.

If we're paying at least twice as much as anyone else on healthcare, and we're not anywhere near the top of healthcare services, *where is all that money going?*

The Promises of Reform

It's not like the government hasn't tried to fix the problem. The following is a list of some major legislation passed by Congress intended to make healthcare more effective and more affordable for the American people. Details on these reforms will be provided in chapter 5.

While some of the names may not be familiar, you have already experienced, unknowingly, difficulties they create when you go to the doctor or to the hospital. So the question really is, why has all this "fixing" of healthcare made things worse?

1965—Medicare, passed into law within the Social Security Act Amendments of 1965

1965—Medicaid was also part of the Social Security Act Amendments and Title XIX

1986—EMTALA, Emergency Medical Treatment and Active Labor Act

1995—UMRA, Unfunded Mandate Reform Act

1996—HIPAA, Health Insurance Portability and Accountability Act

2010—ACA, Patient Protection and Affordable Health Care Act

The latest—the Affordable Care Act (ACA or Obamacare)—promised it would make things better. What has it accomplished for America and for Americans? We will look at the facts, not the hype, in chapter 9.

However, we need to remember *why* President Obama said he needed to reform healthcare. We were spending so much on that system that other vital activities such as infrastructure, education, and the military were suffering from economic starvation. He said we had to "bend down" the spending curve for—reduce national spending on—healthcare.

Despite this very public commitment, the ACA actually has increased U.S. spending on healthcare, and not just a little. Experts estimate that is will cost the inconceivable amount of $2.7 trillion.[2]

The quantity "a trillion dollars" is very hard to comprehend or even to imagine. The figure that follows, adapted from the Internet, may help. In the upper left corner of the illustration, a man is standing next to $1 million dollars, arranged in stacks of one hundred $100 bills ($10,000 in each stack). Look carefully and you will see that the stacks are ten high by ten deep. That is what one million dollars looks like, in $100 bills. For size comparison, the single pallet necessary to support the $1 million is placed next to a man, his leg, actually.

The upper right hand corner of the illustration uses the same concept: stacks of $100 bills, but now each pallet holds $100 million, not one million. It takes ten of those pallets to make up $1 billion.

The lower panel shows what $1 trillion looks like. There are 10,000 double-stacked pallets, with each carrying $100,000,000 (one hundred million dollars!) in $100 bills. The man, for size comparison, is at bottom left.

Every year since 2011, the U.S. has spent well over $2 trillion per year on the healthcare. Approximately $1 trillion went to its bureaucracy and not to health care services or goods for you and me. I had to estimate that number based on my detailed analysis of the federal budget. The government doesn't keep records of its spending on its own bureaucracy (and believe me, I've looked).

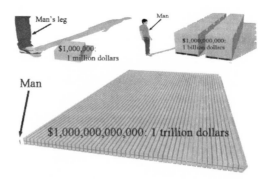

Remember when we used to groan that Ronald Reagan's deficit was going to bankrupt our children? ACA has raised the amount of debt *three times* greater than the amount that Reagan did. No bank on the planet would *ever* loan an individual or even a Fortune 500 company that kind of cash, but the United States borrows it daily.

What this comes down to is that ACA's promised "cost-cutting" is actually spending gargantuan sums of money that we don't have.[3] The table that follows reveals changes in our national debt. A large part of that doubling from 2005 to 2012 is due to ACA. In fact, ACA now holds a new "record" we would rather not have. As a result of President Obama's signature domestic program, ACA, for the first time in our history, starting in 2012, U.S. national debt exceeds our gross domestic product (GDP), in other words, our debt became greater than *all* our productivity!

Is this any way to create a sustainable government and a successful country?

U.S. National Debt Compared to U.S. GDP				
Year	President	National Debt ($$ billions)	GDP ($$ billions)	Debt ÷ GDP
2005	Bush	7,918	12,900	61%
2006	Bush	8,493	13,700	62%
2007	Bush	8,993	14,300	63%
2008	Obama	10,011	14,750	68%
2009	Obama	11,898	14,400	83%
2010	Obama	13,551	14,800	92%
2011	Obama	14,781	15,400	96%
2012	Obama	16,059	16,050	100%*
2013	Obama	16,732	16,600	101%
2014	Obama	17,810	17,250	103%
GDP = Gross Domestic Product. $$=U.S. dollars *=First time in U.S. history				

And here's an even scarier thought: both Congress and the White House have always low-balled the initial estimate of what they would eventually spend on entitlement programs. The year 1990 was the twenty-fifth anniversary of the signing into Law (1965) of Medicare. With twenty-five years of good, hard data in hand, the GAO (Government Accounting Office) compared actual spending to what had been initially projected. The 1965 Congressional estimate missed the actual amount spent by Medicare, by *744 percent*: the predicted cost was $9 billion while the actual cost was $67 billion.[4] When you start with numbers like one trillion and you're off by over seven hundred percent, well, no nation can sustain that kind of mistake. Talk about a national nightmare.

Don't forget President Obama's bold reassurance that, "if you like your doctor, you can keep your doctor" (June 15, 2009).[5] That was just vainglorious. More and more U.S. physicians are quitting. But those numbers aren't being made up in medical school graduates because fewer are becoming doctors. Of those doctors remaining in the profession, more and more cannot afford to accept Medicare or Medicaid reimbursement rates. The cycle is spiraling downward fast.

One of the reasons why so many doctors are quitting is that government payment schedules are so low that your Medicare doctor may be forced to join you in the line of people declaring medical bankruptcy. To avoid closing their practices altogether, doctors are closing their practices to Medicare patients. On July 31, 2013, the *Wall Street Journal* reported that close to ten thousand more doctors opted out of the Medicare program than the prior year.[6] What good is having insurance like Medicare if you can't get medical care?

Oh, and remember those two promised programs I mentioned above: CLASS (supporting seniors) and PCIP (insurance for pre-existing conditions)? Washington has cancelled the former—so much for making sure our grandmothers have long-term disability care—as well as the latter. In February 2013, Washington discontinued enrollment in PCIP when barely 30 percent of those with pre-existing conditions had enrolled, leaving over a quarter of a million of the most fragile and sickliest Americans out in the cold.[7]

The U.S. healthcare system has become an all-too-real nightmare. Our personal dreams have been shattered. Promises made to our nation are starting to look more and more like snake oil.

So I have to ask again: *Where does all that money go?* We're pouring more money into this new system created by ACA than ever before, yet we still cannot get care. Our providers suffer from the burden of over-regulation. In order to support this ever-growing monster called

U.S. healthcare, Washington steals resources from other services, like educating our children.

But here's the truly scary part. The money and the value it represents isn't just disappearing, it is being consumed, eaten up by an entity that, once-upon-a-time, was supposed to help us but instead now serves its own greedy quest for power, an entity that doesn't recognize political boundaries but rather uses all resources available to it at the expense of those it's supposed to serve, We The Patients.

As I said in the introduction, healthcare has cancer, a nasty, nation-eating blight. If you and I do not recognize and accept the diagnosis, the grand idea that is America could, in fact, "perish from the earth."

THREE

Ally to Enemy

Have you been to your doctor lately? If you got in, did she or he have to spend twenty minutes of your thirty-minute appointment filling out forms and asking questions like "Did your mother smoke?" and "What is the level of your pain today?" or "Are you feeling depressed or suicidal?"

I always thought it was surreal to watch my nurse interrogate my six-month old patient (not her mother) "What is your level of pain today?" and "Have you considered suicide lately?" She does this, despite the baby's inability to speak yet, because it is a federal regulation. These are questions that must be asked, by law, of every patient entering the doctor's office. The rule allows no exceptions for age, hearing, or lack of teeth.

The rule that the nurse is following has nothing to do with the baby's health and everything to do with the bureaucracy justifying its existence. It is also part of an effort by the powers-that-be to put more and more personal information into a large national database.

They are stealing your extremely limited time with your doctor in order to collect data that some bureaucrat thought might be useful to him or her. These "regulations" are Washington stealing precious care time—both yours and your health care provider's. But it begs the question: Aren't care providers supposed to care more for you than what some faceless bureaucrat says?

When we go to the doctor, we all have expectations. We expect our doctor to care about us as individuals and about our personal wellbeing. We expect that she or he will perform to the best of his or her training and abilities. We expect, in fact we demand, that we walk away on a path that leads to better health.

We all know that health care hasn't been that way for years. We also know that when our dreams turn into nightmares, we start searching around for someone to blame.

It doesn't seem like we have to search very hard. Because our doctors are the front line, they are the easiest to point a finger at. It's a bitter pill to swallow. We would like to think our personal physician should be our closest ally. Doctors are supposed to take care of us, tell us what's wrong, and give us the right treatment to make us healthy again. They are supposed to "be there" for us no matter what.

But more and more, we have come to distrust the doctors. It seems like they are behaving more and more like an enemy. They have no time for us. They prescribe medicines that drug companies bribe them to give us rather than the ones we really need. To add insult to injury (literally), they get paid tons of money *because* we are sick.

It reminds me of something that happened when I was a kid back in the 1960's. I grew up in a large apartment building in a fancy part of Manhattan. We lived on floor 12AB. The building's elevator designers designated the thirteenth floor as "12AB" because they thought the number thirteen might bring bad luck. On the street level there was a doctor's office. Double-parked outside, waiting for the doctor every morning, was a chauffeur-driven convertible Rolls Royce. (I've always wondered how much that car cost.)

As I have mentioned, I come from a family of doctors. They all made comfortable livings but no one expected to drive a Rolls. I had no clue how a doctor could or would make that kind of money, so I asked my mother about it. (My father died when I was young.)

She smiled with only part of her mouth. "Obviously, you don't know the dark side of medicine," she said. "If a doctor wants to, he can make *a lot* of money."

"How," I asked? "There are only so many patients and so many hours of the day."

"You don't know who that doctor is—" she paused for a moment as if she wasn't sure that she should say anything more but then decided to continue. "That doctor is the Medical Commissioner of the City of New York. When a policeman, firefighter, or sanitation worker is hurt on the job, that doctor decides who gets disability and how much they get. I bet his official salary is $20-30,000 per year [remember, this was in the 1960s], but under the table, he is probably taking ten times that amount."

Obviously, even as a teenager, I knew that $30,000 wasn't *that* much money but $300,000 was. I guess times haven't changed that much.

Even though I don't want to write unkind remarks about my profession, I've seen it play out many times. Part of the greed in healthcare is the unethical doctor who is willing to be bribed—by unscrupulous pharmaceutical companies, unions, and who knows who else. Our system not only allows but sometimes it actively encourages such behavior. Greed is everywhere.

When the government runs the system, the corruption is even more pronounced. GlaxoSmithKline, one of the pharmaceutical giants, was recently accused of bribing doctors in China.[1] Reporters found that such bribery was common practice in China. The government-paid physicians there are paid so poorly that they must accept money "under the table" just so they can eat.

In short, it appears that our oldest healthcare ally, the doctor, is now acting like an adversary. When we are subjected to superfluous but expensive tests; when we are "provided" an excess of services or even unnecessary operations; it doesn't take much to figure out that greed has taken over the management of our care.

Victim and "Perp"

How often do things go wrong during medical care? No doubt you have read some *Reader's Digest* excerpt about things that doctors and nurses do that We The Patients never hear about—like prescribing one medication that combines badly with another the patient is already taking. Together, they create a lethal brew that puts the patient in an emergency department, an ICU bed, or worse, the morgue.

Suppose the treatment just didn't work: You are no worse but your back still hurts. What if, heaven forbid, your mother dies after heart surgery? Do these bad outcomes instantly and automatically turn the doctor into the spawn of the devil?

Doctors are human, and like the rest of us, they make mistakes. Is it right that your relationship with your doctor changes in a blink?

JR (not his real name) is a child I held before his mother did. True, she grew him but she was asleep when he was born and he was immediately transferred to our hospital for care of his quite obvious heart problem. Mother would proudly remind JR that I kissed him before she did.

We fixed his heart problem at two days of age. After the operation, we had to put in a pacemaker to control his heart rhythm. That all worked well and he did fine over several years. He needed a battery change for his pacemaker when he was four years old, no problem.

At age fifteen, JR needed another pacemaker change. I referred the boy (now bigger than I am) to an electrophysiology (EP) specialist, someone who deals only with heart rhythm problems. That doctor operated, removing the old pacemaker and putting in a new one, which worked fine.

Two weeks later, while the EP surgeon was out of the state on vacation, JR developed an infection. He had to go back to the operating room to take out the infected pacemaker. And during that operation, the new surgeon found that the first surgeon had left a piece of gauze under the newly implanted device. That caused the infection.

After antibiotics cleared up the infection, another new pacemaker was inserted surgically in a different location. It worked fine. JR is now back to normal.

When the first surgeon heard about the infection, he cut his vacation short and came home. He tried to talk with and apologize to the mother, but she would not speak with him.

JR's mother did have more than a few words to share with me about the first surgeon. Most of them I cannot write here. The family filed a lawsuit against the first surgeon and the hospital, which is currently pending trial.

Where one month ago, the first surgeon had been her son's savior, now he was the Prince of Darkness. Amazing, isn't it, how quickly relationships can change.

Postscript: Before I retired, I visited with JR and his family. The family was sad. JR gave me a big hug then stepped back and put both hands on the sides of my face. He studied me intently for at least thirty seconds, withdrew his hands and asked, "Why are you retiring? You've got a few good years left!"

The current healthcare system has allowed the patient/doctor relationship to become completely lopsided. The doctor is always and immediately the perpetrator, the one "who done me wrong." The patient is of course the victim. When you have that dynamic at play, things go downhill fast. Our old ally, the doctor, is magically transformed into a "perp." Now we are victims of an evil person. We expect compensation and justice for those who hurt us.

The immediate result is loss of confidence: we no longer trust our doctors.

Without trust, how can any doctor give us the best care possible?

Here Comes the Ambulance Chaser

When a patient does not do well in our current healthcare world, the doctor and deep-pocket hospital are automatically *guilty until proven innocent*. The potential for really big money arises, and in swoops the negligence lawyer. With his encouragement, the patient begins to dream of winning lottery numbers.

Often called "ambulance chasers," these are men (mostly male) who grandly promise you a huge settlement from that negligent S.O.B. who hurt you. It doesn't matter that the same S.O.B. just yesterday was your long-time, reliable friend and trusted healer.

Of course, these ambulance chasers have your best interest at heart. They only want justice done for you and to the doctor. The 40 percent fee they will get has nothing to do with it. (I write this paragraph with tongue firmly in cheek.)

"Obviously," your negligence lawyer assures you, "the doctor *and* the hospital messed up. Their negligence caused your injuries. No question about it." As you happily sign the lawsuit papers you may not even notice the inclusion of "hospital" in the conversation. They're the ones with the big bucks, the ones the lawyer will collect from. I know. I've been at the short end of that stick.

> E.M was a nine-year old swimming in a race when all of a sudden she stopped swimming and went flaccid in the pool. Her coach jumped in, fished her out, and did CPR, bringing her back from sudden cardiac arrest.
>
> Her family brought her to me for consultation at the large university hospital in Chicago where I was Chief of Pediatric Cardiology. I could find absolutely nothing wrong at that time. I therefore had to assume that she had had a sudden, near-fatal heart rhythm disturbance. For this reason, I started her on a medicine to reduce irritability in the heart. She tolerated the drug without problem and had no further incidents.
>
> After seven months of traveling a long distance to see me periodically, the family called to say that they had decided to change physicians to a more convenient one. He was an excellent doctor who worked at the small community hospital near their home. The new doctor reviewed the records, thought everything was okay, but lowered the dosage of the medication a little bit.

The child continued to do well for another five months. Then her older brother found her dead in her bed while the parents were dining out. No cause of death was definitely determined. It was (again) assumed that she had a heart-rhythm issue.

The family sued me and the large University Hospital as well as the other doctor and his small hospital. The jury found for the plaintiff. They awarded the family $8 million to come from the deep-pocket "rich" university. They found me negligent even though I was not even the child's doctor when she died. And for icing on the cake, the jury held the second (treating physician) blameless along with the small (not rich) local, religious-affiliated hospital.

How did I go from being the protector and savior of their precious daughter to the vile perpetrator of her demise—without doing a thing?

One minute the doctor is your most trusted ally and the next, with the medical malpractice (med-mal) lawyer as midwife and new ally, your doctor is reborn as the devil incarnate.

Is the medical negligence lawyer really your ally? Well, he does constantly remind you, "I don't get paid if you don't get paid." (The initial retainer doesn't count.)

The fact of the matter is, the average med-mal lawyer is not involved so you can get a proper compensation or to achieve a just and honorable result. He is playing a game. You are merely a player, admittedly an important one, in a winner-take-all competition, where "all" can be millions of dollars.

The entire medico-legal system is based on tort law, which makes it strictly an adversarial contest. Tort law comes from ancient times where there was trial by combat. It is now used in civil court to provide relief for persons who have suffered because of the wrongful acts of others.

Tort systems are designed to do two things: Identify the perpetrator and "make whole" the victim. That's it. The plaintiff is the patient: he or she is the one who has sustained injury. The defendant is the doctor, nurse, medical group, hospital, and sometimes a medical manufacturer. They are the persons presumably responsible for inflicting the injury. This train wreck is moved along nicely by the plaintiff's negligence lawyer and by the defendant's multitude of high-priced lawyers. I'm sure you can see how easily this system can be manipulated.

Learning from what happened to the patient; doing better in the future; even avoiding a repetition of the incident, NONE of these is an intended outcome of our current system.[2] Money is.

Second, your negligence lawyer—the ambulance chaser—is there solely to win. Truth is irrelevant. As they say in the movie *Michael Clayton*, "The truth can be adjusted." Cause and effect are immaterial. Logic fades under the onslaught of emotion, usually anger. Appearance is everything. The more a med-mal lawyer can create sympathy, the bigger the award or the quicker the settlement. Cases involving facial injuries or children are the best, from the viewpoint of a plaintiff's lawyer.

I well remember a case that I summed up in my notes with four words. They were the reason that the defendant's insurance company settled for a very large sum of money and fast. The defense lawyers never seriously considered going to trial. They didn't care about the reality of who did what or who didn't do what. They knew that perception was key.

The four words were: "Drunk nurse; Dead baby." Got the picture? See why this was settled almost immediately?

In the both of the cases above, the reasoning, such as it was, seemed straightforward. "Children shouldn't die, ever! When they do, someone must have made a terrible mistake.[3] The family must be compensated for their loss. Let's make someone pay, someone who can certainly afford it."

Baby TC was born prematurely but at a good weight of three and a half pounds. He spent sixteen days in the hospital, never on a ventilator, and went home growing nicely on no medications. He became a normal healthy child.

A few months after his second birthday, TC contracted a viral infection called RSV (respiratory syncytial virus). He was seen in a local hospital ER, given some medications and sent home. He was sleeping peacefully in his bed at 4:00 a.m. when he father came in from work.

At 7:30 a.m., when his mother checked on him, TC was not breathing, cold, and dead.

The autopsy protocol said that the TC died because of the RSV infection. It should have read "with" not "because of" RSV: the precise reason why the child died was never found. Because the autopsy used the phrase "because of," the family's lawyer felt a case could be made that the hospital ER should have admitted the child and he would then have survived.

(Keep in mind that to this very day, we do not know why TC died, so how could anyone be sure he would *not* have died in the hospital? Do people never die in hospital?)

The family sued. To shorten a long and most unpleasant story, you can guess what happened. The hospital calculated costs under various scenarios and took the cheapest course: they settled. In fact, no one did anything wrong. Nonetheless, the child was declared a victim of medical negligence. The doctor and the hospital were *therefore* labeled negligent providers. In other words, they became "perps."

In the current system, doctors can't win. They practice defensive medicine and are still painted as wrongdoers even when they do nothing wrong. If they don't order that medically "unnecessary" head scan, they cannot defend themselves in court. If they do, they are padding the bill.

Many doctors try to avoid the most complex, sickest patients, who have the highest likelihood of bad outcomes and may be the most litigious. Of course, these are the same patients who need well-trained, conscientious, and experienced doctors the most.

Doctors pay outrageous malpractice insurance premiums because the system is so complex and flawed. And who pays those costs? Patients do, eventually.

The question that patients must ask themselves is this: When something bad happens during medical care, should that bad thing instantly change your relationship with your doctor? Is the immediate rush to see a negligence lawyer in your best interest? You may win a decent settlement but end up paying higher insurance premiums and doctor fees. Then, good luck trying to find a new doctor who will take you.

Like the rest of healthcare, the medico-legal system is broken. If we would ever discuss it, and Lord knows we should, there are a number of matters on which we all agree. There is one big question where I doubt we have consensus.

We all want patients who suffer avoidable medical injuries to get help and to get compensation. We all concur, except probably for the Trial Lawyers Association, that compensation should go to the injured, not to the ambulance chaser.

We all agree that physicians who are truly negligent, not those who simply made an understandable error in judgment, should be punished in some way.

Everyone wants medical science to learn from things that go wrong so they won't happen in the future. In other words, we want a system that can give us better medical outcomes in the future than it can provide today.

What we may not agree on is what to do with a patient who is injured through no one's fault. The story of one of my favorite patients will illustrate.

In 1999, a young man, "Chuck" (not his real name), walked into my office. He was critically ill with a condition called PPH, primary pulmonary hypertension. Despite his total exercise intolerance, forty-plus pound weight gain, and taunting at school because he was so "fat," he still had a positive attitude. (That is partly why I liked him so much.)

There is no cure for PPH. To this day, we do not know what causes it. There was (and is) an extremely expensive treatment called Prostacyclin®, which can reduce the symptoms. After doing the necessary confirmatory tests, I began the treatment and Chuck improved. Three months later, during one of his routine visits, he proudly informed me that, "he cost his dad a hell of a lot of money." He was not referring to the $10,000/month for the medicine, which he did not know about. Chuck had lost all that extra weight, forty pounds of water, and his dad had to buy him a whole new wardrobe, he explained, grinning.

After three years of taking the medicine, Chuck suddenly became sick with an overwhelming infection. He died less than forty-eight hours after the fever started. One of the known side effects of Prostacyclin is to reduce the body's ability to fight infection.

Should the medico-legal system compensate the family for this worst of all possible outcomes? Should it not? Should patients be compensated for all adverse outcomes, even when the cause of the injury is unknown and even when there is no evidence of negligence? In Chuck's case, no one did anything wrong. His death was a terrible but unavoidable tragedy. Nonetheless, a child died during medical care.

There is an alternative to our current medico-legal system suggested in the Appendix titled "Fixing Medical Malpractice." Read it and see what you think.

The Fallacy of the Efficient Doctor

Believe it or not, "efficiency" is one of the main reasons why health care service stinks. If that strikes you as odd, join the club. We think we want our doctors to be efficient. Hospitals and managers expect, in fact they demand, that doctors be efficient. What you and I don't know is that "efficient" has become the polite term for complying with regulations and spending as little time as possible with the patient.

I remember my own pediatrician quite clearly—Dr. Schneck. He always smelled funny, at least to me as a young boy. I think it was from disinfectant. He was consistently nice to me and spent a lot of time talking with my mother. I wasn't sick that often as a child. I did have behavioral problems, probably related to my dysfunctional family and the fact that my father died suddenly and very unexpectedly when I was fourteen.

My mother and I spent quite a lot of time talking with Dr. Schneck. Whether he actually did something to make me healthier, or simply made my mother feel better by listening, I do not know. Regardless, what he did then does not happen in today's healthcare world. It is actively discouraged.

"Efficient" literally means more work per unit time. In other words, an efficient doctor sees more patients per day than an inefficient one. Obviously, the more efficient the doctor is, the less time she or he has with any one patient. Efficiency (less time with each patient) is rewarded; inefficiency (spending more time with patients) is punished.

According to national standards, I am supposed to see 4.2 "established" (not new) patients per hour. That means one every *fourteen* minutes.

I am a pediatric cardiologist. Most of my patients are babies and small children. Before you can even try to examine one of my patients, you have to make friends with him or her. That takes time. Getting the history from the young and frightened mother takes time. Explaining congenital heart problems takes lots of time, including drawing pictures of a normal heart and then the child's abnormal heart. I *never* could do all that in fourteen minutes or even thirty minutes. I usually took forty-five minutes to an hour to see a patient.

By definition, I was very inefficient. If I had continued practicing medicine that way, both my hospital and I would have been penalized for it.

And here's the really sad part. Guess who bears the brunt of those penalties for "inefficiency"? You do.

If you want time to talk with your health-care provider, you cannot have that with an "efficient" doctor. The system forces your doctor to deny you the very thing you want, expect, and need.

It is just more proof that the cancer has spread to the very core of the healthcare system: The doctor-patient connection. Your doctor probably does care about you. She or he wants to help you get better but doctors are at the mercy of the healthcare (one word) system, which is controlled by the cancer. It could care less about you. Rather it licks its greedy lips as you're admitted to the doctor's office because it knows how much it's going to make off of you.

Natural Enemies?

This leads me to ask a question I never dreamed I would ever ask. In this brave new world of ACA healthcare, is it possible that providers and patients have become "natural enemies"? That would be truly terrifying.

If doctors and patients are now natural adversaries, the doctor-patient relationship becomes one of predator (provider) to prey (you). If this is true, healthcare is more than just hazardous to your health. It could be lethal.

Natural enemies are lions and gazelles on the African savannah, or hawks and mice in your own back yard—the classic predator and prey scenario.

Natural predators survive by eating their prey. In the predator–prey relationship, the predator does well when the prey does … poorly.

If you become sick, the doctor has work to do and gets paid. The sicker you are, the more the provider must do and thus, the more she or he gets paid. I am sure you have heard the term "pay for performance." In essence, this is a predator-prey relationship. The provider "preys" on the sickly patient. The doctor or hospital does better the sicker you are.

It's not hard to see why this happens. How many times has your doctor ordered an expensive CT scan or MRI for something that seemed to be rather minor? Is it because they're being thorough or are they CYA (Covering Your Anatomical-posterior part), using your money? How many of these questionable tests are ordered because the healthcare system needs to CYA, and the doctors are just following "instructions" (you can call them federal guidelines)?

Healthcare providers are paid based on how much they perform. The more they do *for* us (or should I write *to* us?), the more money they make. Or at least that's what it appears to be on the surface.

When I was a small child, I frequently visited and stayed with my grandparents in Brooklyn. My grandfather was a physician. In his day, doctors were either physicians or surgeons. That's it. There was no such thing as specialists, much less subspecialists like me. Grandfather Michael took care of everyone. That is what physicians did in his day.

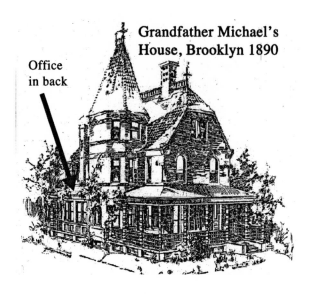

Office in back

Grandfather Michael's House, Brooklyn 1890

I loved to sneak in to his office, which was attached to the big house, but which had a separate entrance. I would hide and watch what he did. This would be absolutely against current confidentiality rules. I hope the statute of limitations has run out for confidentiality infractions I was guilty of more than sixty years ago.

I remember a conversation I overheard between my grandfather and his nurse that, sadly, would never happen today. An elderly patient had come in with chest pain and my grandfather examined him. Dr. Michael—that is what everyone called my grandfather—gave the patient a piece of paper (a prescription for antibiotics) and asked him to come back the following day. On the way out, Mr. X took out his wallet and carefully gave the nurse/receptionist two slightly crumpled dollar bills to pay for his visit with Dr. Michael.

After the patient left, my grandfather said to the nurse, "I think Mr. X has pneumonia but I'm not sure. He certainly cannot afford to be in the hospital and probably can't even pay for a chest x-ray. So, I asked him to come back tomorrow so I can listen again to his lungs. Let's not charge him for that."

Can you imagine this scenario playing out in today's world of healthcare? Not a chance! What has changed is that greed is in charge, cancer is in control, not you and not your physician.

Though finger pointers love to blame the doctors for all the problems we experience trying to get health care, the fact is that the system is the problem: chaotic, confusing, contradictory, and not designed to help us.

Doctor, Replaced

As we have seen, there are a number of different possible doctor-patient relationships in healthcare today. There is also the absence of one—no relationship. If there is one major culprit in the nightmare that we call healthcare, it is when the doctor cannot practice medicine because he or she has been replaced.

With the development of the third-party payer system (another name for insurance) and increasingly stringent government control of medicine, the physician is, simply, being taken out of the healthcare equation.

Here's the hard truth: *Doctors have been replaced by bureaucrats, both corporate as well as government.*

The bureaucrat is the puppeteer, the person behind the scenes making up the rules of the game, changing the goal lines and the yard markers.

Several years ago, a baby girl (YM) was born to a young Hispanic couple as their first child. Baby Y was beautiful and instantly captivated her father, as girl babies tend to do. (Mine certainly did forty-odd years ago.)

Baby Y had a complex congenital heart problem where the two major blood vessels were in the wrong place, and there was a big hole between the pumping chambers.[4] We had not had good results with repair of this problem at my own institution and had stopped doing the operation many years ago. We sent these patients to other centers.

As part of our care for patients, we had reviewed all the results from many centers around the U.S. and found one with the best outcomes by far. Let's call it hospital A.

I told the parents all this and recommended that we send the child to hospital A. They concurred.

Baby Y was covered by Medicaid, the government-provided health insurance program for children. The insurance carrier that had the Medicaid contract for our region said they had a formal commitment with hospital B. That is where she must go for surgery. I shared outcomes' data with the medical director that showed how much better hospital A's outcomes were compared to hospital B's. He was unmoved. He repeated that my patient had to go to hospital B. With great trepidation, I sent her there.

A predictable, avoidable tragedy unfolded.

At three weeks of age, the team at hospital B repaired her heart. However, there was damage to the diaphragm, the muscle that controls breathing. They could not remove her from the mechanical ventilator until she had a second operation to repair her diaphragm.

During a prolonged stay in the ICU (several weeks), baby Y gradually developed a blockage inside her heart where a patch of material had been placed. As this became severe, a third operation was required. They took out the first patch and put in another one. After this procedure, the baby had damage to the conduction system in her heart and needed a pacemaker placed (operation number four).

She remained quite ill in the hospital and needed a cardiac catheterization to sort out what was happening. It became clear that one of the valves inside her heart—the mitral—had been damaged at operation number three and was failing. It had to be repaired. That required heart surgery number five at the age of four months.

Unfortunately, she was worse after this procedure. An echocardiogram showed that the mitral valve still leaked a lot but now the aortic valve leaked as well, presumably injured at operation #5. Her sixth surgery was a repair of the aortic valve and re-repair of the mitral. After this, she slowly recovered and was discharged on four different medications having spent over five months in the Intensive Care Unit (at more than $5000/day).

If the recommendations of her doctor (that's me) had been followed, Baby Y would have gone to the hospital that had the best results. She would have had one surgery, spent about two weeks in hospital, and required one medication after surgery. The total cost would have been approximately $75, 000.

Instead, her insurance "doctor"—a bureaucrat with neither an MD degree nor medical training other than billing—replaced me. He (actually she) had the final say, and sent my patient to hospital B. There, baby Y was subjected to six surgeries, spent the first five months of life in an ICU bed, and still has major residual heart disease that will require even more surgery later. Her hospital bill was in excess of $2 million.

If you detect a hint of anger in my recounting of this story, you are right. It is there, in full force. She is still a beautiful little girl, but she has trouble walking and speaking because of brain damage from those early events.

You, as patient, no longer get to decide what the best care is for you. Neither does your doctor—and that should terrify you.

I certainly had no control over the care of "my" patient, YM. Doctors are supposed to be in control of their patient's care. Since I wasn't, who was? Who decided the best way to care for her? The insurance company's bureaucrat thought that she should decide because her company was footing the bill. What a bunch of hogwash!

Like most of you, YM's parents had dutifully paid into the insurance system every month so that when a catastrophe occurred, they or their child would receive the best care possible. But because the insurance company was in charge of the bills, the insurance agent figured that she should be the one telling the doctor how to practice medicine. How is that right?

By now, you are probably asking yourself, why do nurses and doctors put up with it? Many don't because they have come to the stark realization that every minute of every day millions of American health care providers must face the following:

- Medical problems for which there are no good—safe and effective—treatments, yet patients expect doctors to have perfect solutions for every ailment
- Non-compliant patients, consumers, or clients
- Mind-numbing, time-sucking, impossible-to-do-right bureaucratic red tape
- Devaluation of providers' services by payers and administrators
- Guilty until proven innocent: The automatic presumption that the provider is at fault whenever a patient suffers a bad outcome
- The constant (losing) battle with insurance carriers to get patients the care they need
- A system that is supposed to help providers offer health care, but obstructs them at every turn.

Put yourself in your doctor's shoes. Think about waking up every day of your working life knowing that you must face the list above.

Before I retired, I started to ask myself these questions every day: "Why do I put up with this? Why do I keep banging my head against a brick wall? I have skills and education. There are lots of other things I can do for more money and much, much less aggravation." I never seemed to find a satisfactory explanation why I stayed in clinical practice. Then, one day, I found it.

The Head Nurse where I worked is a bulwark of the division. She knows everyone and everything, including how to get around the rules so patients can get what they need. She has two children in college and an almost five-year-old "surprise" named Jonah.

The nurse also has a chronic medical condition and occasionally can be quite ill. Nonetheless, she is highly conscientious and always calls in when she cannot come in to the office.

One day she failed to show up for work and there was no explanatory call. Becoming concerned, I speed-dialed her cell phone and got a whispering child who was certainly Jonah.

"Hello," he said softly.

"Jonah," I replied, "Is your mom at home?"

"Yes," whispered the small voice.

"May I talk with her?"

The child whispered, "No."

Surprised and wanting to make sure she was okay, I asked, "Jonah, is your dad there?"

"Yes."

"May I talk with him?"

Again Jonah's small voice softly said, "No."

Getting frustrated, I asked, "Is anybody else there?"

"Yes," whispered the child, "some policemen."

Wondering why the police were there, I asked, "May I speak with one of them?"

"No, you can't. They're busy," he answered.

"Busy doing what?"

"Talking to Mommy and Daddy, ... and the Fireman."

Hearing a loud background noise through the phone, I asked with some real concern, "What is that noise?"

"A helicopter," answered the still whispering child.

"What the hell is going on?" I demanded.

"The search team just landed in a helicopter."

Now truly terrified, I shouted, "What are they searching for?"

The young voice replied with a muffled giggle ... "*Me.*"

Regardless of how much fun we doctors might have treating our individual patients, doctor-patient relationships have become strained. The practice of medicine has become painful. No, it is worse than that. Dr. Ed Marsh explained it well in the *Wall Street Journal* where he explained why he "couldn't take it anymore." Dr. Marsh is now an _ex_-physician; he retired early from clinical practice because, as he wrote, "The glow of the personal relationship one might have with one's patients is being [actively] extinguished."[5]

Whatever name you use—doctor, physician, health care delivery person, predator, perp—these are the people who used to be your friends and allies. They are gone. They have been replaced by bureaucrats. Your new "doctors" are solely concerned with themselves and sadly, they care not a whit about you or your health.

Who are these greedy S.O.B.s? We need to keep in mind sage advice from over 2500 years ago: Know thy enemy (Sun Tzu.)

FOUR

Faces of Greed

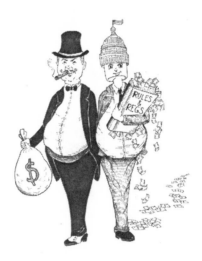

G reed has many faces. Two are our enemies in healthcare. They are symbolized above. In my mind, they are Siamese twins joined at the hip, or more accurately, joined at the hip pocket where they keep their wallets.

On the right is a representation of a greedy government bureaucrat with his head made of the Capitol Dome. A good friend of mine claims no such person exists. In chapter 6, we will consider whether the greedy government bureaucrat is a figment of my imagination or is real.

On the left is the private or corporate symbol of greed. I modeled him after the moustache-sporting, top hat wearing "Monopoly Man," who has been the marketing icon for the famous Parker board game,

Monopoly.[1] In this chapter, we will investigate the real world faces of corporate greed in healthcare.

There is solid evidence to believe that corporate greed contributes to our problems in getting health care. I've already told you about a few of the run-ins I have had with insurance companies. There were hundreds of such painful interactions. It got to the point where I couldn't take it anymore.

I was livid because I felt that all those years I studied, trained, and used my knowledge and skills helping patients, were being wasted. Instead, I was forced to spend more and more time fighting verbally with Medical Directors of insurance conglomerates who don't give a da*n if my patients live or die. I retired soon after the following incident:

> A baby with a very abnormal heart was the first child born to young Spanish-speaking parents. Uncorrected, the malformation would soon cause the baby to die.
>
> One surgeon (Dr. X) who was twelve hundred miles away had experimented with special repair techniques. He had developed a way to fix the baby's problem in one operation.
>
> I tried to send the baby to Dr. X. The insurance company said they had a contract with a different but widely respected surgeon (Dr. Y) and that I had to send the baby to him.
>
> I called Dr. Y and discussed the baby with him. "Of course I can do the surgery," he said without hesitation. He went on to explain that he was comfortable with the old, partial, now-obsolete technique.
>
> I then called back the Medical Director of the insurance company and showed him data proving that Dr. X and the technique he developed was the best, the right, indeed the only, choice for this baby. I said that Dr. Y was not an acceptable alternative. The Director was unmoved. "The baby goes where we say she goes. After all, we are paying the bill!"

The baby, though stable, had to stay in the hospital because she needed a medicine that could only be given intravenously (IV). It did not work orally.

Administrative battle lines were drawn. The parents and I were on one side: the insurance company was on the other. We considered a lawsuit to compel insurance to send the baby to Dr. X but knew that would take years. I thought about threatening to hold a nasty press conference for the 11:00 p.m. TV news.

Meanwhile, the father did some investigating. He found that he could change insurance carriers to one that would send the baby to Dr. X. However, he could only change the insurance if the baby were discharged from hospital. This meant I would have to stop the life-protecting IV medicine.

After more phone calls, emails, threats, stonewalling, and no progress, I decided I had to take a chance. I stopped the medicine, and discharged the child so the father could change insurance. We made plans to see the baby in my office first thing the next morning. While I was doing this, nursing staff reported me to Hospital Risk Management and to the Chair of my Department.

Next came the irate phone calls from hospital lawyers and the Chairperson warning me about the legal risk that I was creating for myself, my Department, and the hospital by discharging the patient. (The lawyers and administrators didn't understand I *had* to do what was medically dangerous. Otherwise, she would be operated by Dr. Y, which was more dangerous.)

The morning after discharge, the baby was worse. I immediately put her back in the hospital and restarted the medicine she needed. During her eighteen hours at home, her father had been able to switch insurance carriers. I called the Medical Director of the new insurance company and convinced him that the baby should go to Dr. X.

In the neonatal intensive care unit, with the life-saving medicine re-started, the baby returned to a good condition. When I was discussing with the neonatal doctor all the details of transfer to Dr. X's institution, she commiserated with me about everything I had gone through to get the baby the care she needed. (It was the hot topic all over the hospital.) The mother was behind a curtain but heard every word the other doctor said to me.

I went to check on the baby just before the transport team left. The mother came up to me with tears in her eyes. She put her hand on my shoulder and with a shaky voice in broken English, she said, "Thank you for fighting for my baby."

While this father kept his wits and found a way to get his baby the right care, there are many who are not so lucky. Take the case of Deamonte Driver. He died shortly after New Year's Day 2007 when he was twelve years old.[2] If the U.S. healthcare system were not riddled with cancer, he would be in school right now or maybe out playing basketball.

Deamonte was a previously healthy Maryland boy who began complaining of a toothache. His family was poor and though they qualified for Medicaid, he did not see a dentist. Very few local dentists would accept Medicaid reimbursement schedules. Between lack of available providers and administrative delays, Deamonte did not get medical care until he had a seizure and was admitted as an emergency to the hospital.

Five weeks later, after two surgeries and over a quarter of a million dollars in bills, Deamonte died from his brain abscess, a recognized and preventable complication of an infected tooth cavity!

If Medicaid were effective insurance, it would have led to timely healthcare for this boy. If Deamonte had received timely health care, he would be alive today. End of story.

Insurance

The greed exhibited by insurance companies is awe-inspiring. Check out the tallest buildings in New York, Atlanta, Chicago, and San Francisco. Who owns them? Answer: Insurance companies, with their names emblazoned in letters ten feet tall.

In 2010, who was the highest paid CEO in the United States? Answer: Stephen J. Hemsley, CEO of UnitedHealth Group. His salary was $101,960,000, plus unpublished bonuses and benefits (unpublished because if we knew, there would probably be rioting in the streets.)

While the insurance companies are making massive profits, what is happening to us? Like Deamonte's parents, you may not be able to afford health insurance, so you rely on Medicaid, but you can't find a doctor who will accept that form of paltry insurance. You have a good job with benefits, but insurance premiums are going up, up, up, and you wonder how long you will be able to afford your insurance at all. Then you find out that your neighbor had to have chemotherapy and was forced to declare medical bankruptcy, even though she had health insurance.[3] Those are just anecdotes. What is happening to us as a nation? What is happening to We The Patients?

First, note what was happening before Obamacare in the chart that follows.[4] The data was generated by the Kaiser Family Foundation, one of the few sources of data on healthcare that is accurate and reliable. (What makes them reliable is their objectivity and lack of party affiliation. Kaiser Research Foundation is dedicated to solving healthcare problems, not following either Democrat or Republican dogma.)

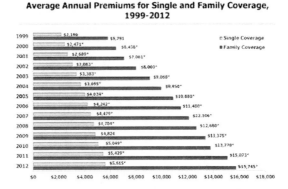

Average Annual Premiums for Single and Family Coverage, 1999-2012

From 1999 to 2012, the average annual cost of individual health insurance premiums rose from $2196 to $5615. For a family of four, the cost of health insurance increased from $5791 to $15,745. Over those thirteen years, that represents a 271 percent increase in cost. I don't know anyone who over the same time period who experienced those levels of pay increases over the same time period. Quite the opposite!

Fifteen thousand, seven hundred and forty-five dollars a year clearly was "unaffordable" health insurance. That is what Obamacare was supposed to fix. Did it?

As you can see in the chart below,[5] President Obama's reform *raised* the average monthly cost of premiums across the board, for all groups. What was unaffordable before ACA is now even more unaffordable. (I know that is not proper grammar but it still sounds right.)

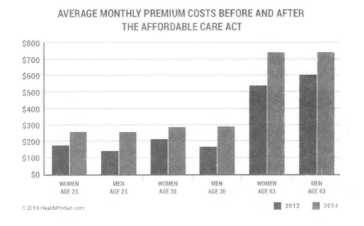

AVERAGE MONTHLY PREMIUM COSTS BEFORE AND AFTER THE AFFORDABLE CARE ACT

So at the same time as Americans were losing their jobs, being converted from fulltime to part-time employees, and watching their paychecks go down, Obamacare was driving the cost of health insurance up and adding new taxes to boot. We have been hit with a double whammy.

Before Obamacare was passed, the number of uninsured Americans was estimated to be between forty-five and fifty million. It became one of the main drivers for passage of the ACA. The excessive expense of insurance was cited as the most common reason why people had no coverage. What the media failed to report and our honored congressmen and women failed to make clear was that twelve to fifteen million uninsured Americans did qualify for Medicaid but chose not to sign up, even though it was free to them. If that doesn't make you ask some hard questions, I don't know what will.

I've already talked about the thirty million Americans who are *under*insured, and I've watched too many families suffer financial hardship because of it. It's a "damned if you have it, damned if you don't" scenario. You pay exorbitant premiums every month. You get sick. You still have to pay impossibly high deductibles, and then you find out you're still not adequately covered. Why bother with insurance at all?[6]

Jeffrey Pfeffer at Harvard, a widely respected management expert and author, recently wrote that insurance companies have "few incentives … to stop wasting their and everyone else's time."[7] With great respect for Professor Pfeffer, he is dead wrong. Insurance companies have a very powerful incentive to waste your time. The longer they delay, defer, or deny your care, the longer they hold on to your money. They are not wasting their time at all. When they say no to you; when they say you filled out the wrong forms; or when they put your doctor's recommendations Under Review, they are making money!

Insurance is alive and doing very well, thank you very much, while we are getting sicker, and then going bankrupt trying to pay the co-pays and the deductibles. Greed pays very well. Mr. Hemsley probably bought a third summer home, this one in Belize.

Big Pharma

Starting in 1997, advertisements for prescription drugs on television have increasingly become more prominent. That's because in that year, the Federal Drug Administration changed their rules for informing consumers about the side effects of drugs.[8] All of a sudden, we're being bombarded with everything from "little purple pills" for indigestion to very dangerous anti-depressant drugs—drugs whose side effects include "liver or heart failure, even death and sometimes suicide." Now you can go to your doctor demanding a certain kind of "miracle" drug because you "saw it on T.V." Drug company profits soared even higher than before, and big pharma became a close second to insurance companies as favorite villain status.

Big pharma is a phrase that lumps all the major pharmaceutical companies together. All are multinationals in the top five hundred of largest corporations in the world according to Fortune magazine. Over half (seven out of twelve) are based in the U.S.

For a sense of magnitude, the following table shows what the "big" means in big pharma. No other product-making industry comes close to big pharma's average profit margin of 19 percent. For comparison, the average profit margin in the oil & gas industry is 6.2 percent.

Most Profitable Pharmaceutical Companies (2014)			
Company name	**Country**	*Net* **Income***	**Profit**
Sanofi-Aventis	France	9.0	13%
AstraZeneca	U.K./Sweden	8.4	17%
Pfizer	U.S.	22.0	17%
Abbott Laboratories	U.S.	2.6	17%
Bayer	Germany	4.7	19%
Roche	Switzerland	12.6	19%
GlaxoSmithKline	U.K.	8.0	19%
Novartis	Switzerland	9.3	20%
Johnson & Johnson	U.S.	13.8	20%
Merck	U.S.	4.4	33%
(*) In billions of U.S. dollars. U.S.=United States. U.K.=United Kingdom.			

It looks like Big Pharma is getting very rich off of our misery and sickness. They *do well* when we *don't*. If they're making that much money, it's a safe bet that we are not doing well health-wise.

If we take things down from the 35,000-foot view to the plight of you and me, things look even worse. Down in the trenches, we have to take out a second (or heaven forbid a third) mortgage to pay for our prescription drugs.

At Walgreen's, here are the prices for a one-month supply of medications whose names you hear advertised on TV. Many people take multiple medications. It's no wonder some people are forced to choose between paying for medicines and buying food.

- Losartan—$88/month (for high blood pressure)
- Lipitor—$241/month (lowers cholesterol; generic form is approximately $100/mo)
- Avelox—$300/month (3rd generation form of Cipro, the famous anti-anthrax drug)
- Flovent—$212/month (for asthma)
- Advair—$280/month (also for asthma)
- Nexium—$245/month ("the little purple pill" for people with stomach acid)
- Cyclosporin—$332/mo (anti-rejection or anti-autoimmune disease)
- Tacrolimus—$272/month (anti-rejection or anti-autoimmune disease)

Say you fall off your bicycle and hit your head. (You were wearing a helmet, right?) You go to the ER and the doctor says you need a head CT. You know this is expensive but you also know that the machine costs millions. Did you ever think about the stuff they inject into you to make clear pictures, the stuff that makes you hot all over very briefly?

That stuff is called liquid contrast or "dye." You will be billed anywhere from $875 to $1200 for one bottle containing 100cc (3 fluid ounces) of the contrast. Thus, you pay around $1000 to big pharma on top of the thousands of dollars for the technical charge (machine/hospital) and hundreds for the doctor's interpretation fee, all because you caught your front wheel in a crack in the pavement.

Although the above prices seem unreasonable, just wait. As they say on late-night TV ads, "You ain't seen nothin' yet!" Check out a big-ticket item called chemotherapy.

Rituxan is the brand name for chemotherapy drug Rituximab made by Genentech, Inc. It will cost you $5500 for one 660mg injection. Depending on the cancer you have and the protocol you accept, you may need as few as eight injections or as many as forty. That means the cost for just *one* of the many drugs you might need could be $220,000.

A personal friend and neighbor shared with me one of her numerous bills for chemotherapy to treat her cancer of the lymph nodes. (I am very pleased to say she beat the big "C.")

The following bill shows charges for drugs of $12,396.36, and that was for one day! Her treatment was repeated five more times over the next four months.

The total charge for pharmaceuticals alone was $74,378.16. Her insurance paid $53, 585.40 to the pharmacy that sells the drugs. My friend has excellent insurance; her husband owns an insurance company! Even so, she is expected to pay out of pocket $20,792.76 just for her chemotherapy drugs only. This does not include doctor's fees or co-payments for the hospitalizations needed to handle the well-described and all-too-frequent complications of the drugs.

SERVICE INFORMATION

	Service Date	Amount Billed	Not Covered	Covered
NM ONCOL HEMAT CONS LTD				
Provider Patient Account No.:				
Drugs	05-25-12	7210.56		7210.56
Drugs	05-25-12	1412.07	1356.41 (1)	55.66
Injections	05-25-12	940.10	722.30 (1)	217.80
Drugs	05-25-12	128.92	115.32 (1)	13.60
Drugs	05-25-12	94.40		94.40
Injections	05-25-12	33.60	30.60 (1)	3.00
Injections	05-25-12	32.50	23.00 (1)	9.50
Drugs	05-25-12	23.60		23.60
Injections	05-25-12	6.10	4.46 (1)	1.64
Therapy	05-25-12	539.00	275.52 (1)	263.48
Therapy	05-25-12	576.68	143.42 (1)	433.26
Therapy	05-25-12	242.17	59.67 (1)	182.50
Treatment Other	05-25-12	292.38	227.92 (1)	64.46
Injections	05-25-12	277.14	211.81 (1)	65.33
Therapy	05-25-12	587.14	295.03 (1)	292.11
Totals		$12396.36	$3465.46	$8930.90

If that doesn't make you want to throw up, you have a stronger stomach than I do. And, believe it or not, things get even worse.

Health Care Organizations

Have you been to any recently built hospital? Whether you are a patient or a visitor, you can't help but notice some of the parallels to an upscale hotel—expensive tile on the foyer floor, large rooms with high ceilings, big bay windows, luxurious furniture, and all the latest equipment.

Hospitals are big business, very big business. Their wealth goes hand-in-glove with insurance company greed. Look at the salaries of hospital administrators. CEOs and other senior administrative types are paid much, much more than the highest paid doctors. Maybe not as much as insurance executives like Mr. Hemsley, but they certainly do (ahem) very, very well.

At New York's famous Sloan-Kettering Institute, each of six administrators makes over one million dollars a year, not counting their (undisclosed) performance bonuses. At Montefiore Hospital, also in New York, the CEO is paid over $4 million per year, the CFO takes away $3.2 million and the Executive VP a measly $2.2 million. (Maybe I went into the wrong side of medicine when I chose to be a lowly practicing doc instead of a hospital administrator.)

At my alma mater, Yale in New Haven, Connecticut, the former-President of the University, Richard Levin, made $1.8 million a year.[9] The CEO of Yale-New Haven Hospital, who in theory *works for* Levin, made $2.5 million a year, not counting his performance bonuses.

Typically, in small communities, hospitals are the biggest tax revenue generators and the largest employers. Montefiore Hospital, a mid-sized hospital in the Bronx, has an annual budget of $2.6 billion. That makes this one hospital, number 161 in the list of 195 *national* GDPs on earth!

Who do you think pays for all that? You and me, that's who, through those ever-increasing insurance premiums, hidden taxes, etc.

Then there are the charges that we see on our hospital bills. What adjective should I use to describe them? Astronomical? Ludicrous? Obscene? "Unaffordable" seems too tame.

Sheryl S. is a forty-six-year old accountant in Piqua, Ohio. She doesn't have a regular doctor. One Thursday night, she began to have chest pains, a problem she had never had before. She called 911 and the paramedics arrived within twelve minutes. They took her to the regional hospital Emergency Department (ED).

There, she was immediately triaged by a nurse, then examined by an ED doctor. He ordered a number of tests and called for an emergency cardiology consult. The cardiologist drove in from home, consulted, and ordered more tests. She was observed on a cardiac monitor for six hours until the follow up tests came back showing that she had no heart problem but only had acid indigestion (heartburn).

This woman spent a total of just over six hours in ED. The hospital bill was $17,345. The charges included ambulance stabilization & transfer ($1150); nursing services ($3800); an electrocardiogram ($126), chest x-ray ($194), and an echocardiogram ($2715); three troponin levels (to check for heart damage) at $200 each plus other blood tests totaling $1954; disposables ($2130); and other sundries/miscellaneous for over $5000. Oh, that $17,345 bill doesn't even count the two doctors' bills, which totaled $3100. Not bad for a couple of hours' work.

Part of one day's hospital bill from a different patient is shown below.

1/04/11	1	0406462	TUBE CONNECTING STERIL 6FT	27.00
1/05/11	1	3005741	ACCU-CHEX CCRV	18.00
1/05/11	1	3019692	SURGICEL 2X14 STRIP EACH	451.00
1/05/11	1	3005741	ACCU-CHEX CCRV	18.00
1/05/11	1	3005741	ACCU-CHEX CCRV	18.00
1/05/11	1-	3019692	SURGICEL 2X14 STRIP EACH	451.00-
1/05/11	1	3005741	ACCU-CHEX CCRV	18.00
1/05/11	1	3005741	ACCU-CHEX CCRV	18.00
1/05/11	10	2900025	OXYGEN HOURLY	560.00
1/05/11	1	0402230	LEUKINS TUBE SPECIM TRAP	77.00
1/05/11	1	0416826	SET EXTENSION 1-VALVE	

Note the small, almost "niggling" charges. They don't seem like much but they add up. In this emergency visit, the patient had four different blood sugar checks in one day for her diabetes. They are the highlighted "Accu-chex CCRV," which uses a chemically embedded strip inside a handheld device. The disposable strips cost fifty-five cents each if bought online. The tests were billed at $18 each.

The above bill also shows the charge for the required sterile surgical strips on the patient's incision. They come two in a pack and cost about seven bucks at a surgical supply store. The hospital charge for the packet was $451 (upper arrow). The patient also needed oxygen during her first night. The charge (lower arrow) was $560 for ten hours' use of the tank.

When you buy one hundred Tylenol (anti-inflammation) pills at Walmart, the whole bottle cost about $1.50. When you buy *one* Tylenol tablet in the hospital, it costs $1.50.

Healthcare Lobbies

Insurance companies and big pharma are the easy villains, the most obvious places where the cancer is winning. Because they are public companies, their profit margins are open for everyone to see. There is another, well-hidden "winner" who lurks behind the face of corporate greed.

Even as the insurance industry makes out like a bandit, and well before ACA, healthcare in the U.S. was one of the most regulated industries of all. How does the corporate side of healthcare greed deal with the government and all its regulations? Answer: The healthcare lobbyist.

In our capitalist system, one has to pay to protect or expand one's business interests. That is why lobbying is so lucrative, both for lobbyist and for his or her employer. That is also why regular hard-working Americans dislike them so much. Lobbyists have a lot of money and can influence congressional opinion far better than we can. The only thing we can do is vote someone out of office, a powerful tool to be sure, but one that only happens every two years, or four years for the White House. Lobbying goes on all the time. (Why do you think the FDA changed its rules about drug advertising in 1997?)

Between 1998 and 2014, the amounts shown below were spent *lobbying* Congress on the behalf of the following industries. Remember, these expenses have nothing to do with making products or providing services. What kind of profit do you think they are expecting when they pay out these sums to lobbyists?

- Oil and gas $1.4 billion
- Defense and Aerospace $1.6 billion
- Healthcare organizations $6.5 billion.
  This includes insurance companies, hospitals, big pharma, HMOs, doctor groups, nursing homes, and allied health services.

In other words, healthcare organizations spent more than double what oil-&-gas and defense industries spent *combined* on efforts to influence the government. Keep in mind that all three are highly regulated by Washington. Healthcare pays better, which is why healthcare corporations spend so much on their lobbying efforts.

Insurance companies, hospitals, big pharma, lobbyists—they get all the benefit, and who do you think pays that bill? That's right: You and me, We The Patients. The same cancer of greed that is killing us is rewarding the hospitals and other healthcare organizations quite well.

Make no mistake; there is a reason why corporate healthcare is so vilified. They make billions because of our illnesses, and then they have to gall to lobby the government to allow them to bilk us out of even more of our hard-earned cash. As we get sicker and we need more care, we find it harder and harder to pay our medical bills. Relief seems to be a fading dream.

The Worst Villain

We watch our paychecks dwindle. We struggle with rising healthcare costs. We desperately want to find the head evildoer and string him (or her) up from the nearest tree. It certainly would feel good. It might even be just. So, which of the culprits listed above is the main villain? Insurance companies? Doctors? Hospitals? Big pharma? Who is ultimately responsible for our nightmares?

The gargantuan over-spending on lobbying gives us our first hard clue. There is something going on in all those regulations that prompt the corporate side of healthcare to spend an inordinate amount to protect its interests.

That ain't right, if you know what I mean.

Have you ever noticed that when people band together in a group, they tend to lose their ability to think rationally as individuals? It's a phenomenon called "groupthink," and it's the reason why our Founding Fathers chose a representative republic, not a democracy, as the basis of our great nation. Groupthink (more on this later) is also known as "mob mentality." People follow what the group is doing, and individual responsibility for decisions and actions quickly goes by the wayside.

Cancer has taken over the entire healthcare system. The cancer is everywhere, with its greedy little fingers in every creviche, taking over everything. Individuals are acting the way the cancer tells them to, not using their own minds. The cancer in healthcare is no longer just the insurance company, a local pharmaceutical rep, that no-time-for-you doctor, or the hospital Medical Director. It's everyone who allows such a system to exist, including the one entity that's supposed to be protecting us from this abuse, the government.

But "therein lies the rub," as Shakespeare wrote.[10] If the government is making the rules, then how much is the government responsible for the continuing success of the cancer?

Let's recap what we know: because of an ever-growing cancer, you have ceased to be a sick person in need of health care. You (patient) are now a *revenue source* for doctor and hospital; a consumer of big pharma products; and an *expense item* for insurance. But maybe what's most disturbing of all is that you are a *vote-for-sale* in Washington.

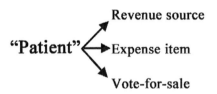

The cancer in our healthcare system has stripped us of our humanity. It has changed us from patients into objects. As a patient myself, I most emphatically resent losing my status as a human being and becoming a revenue source. Professionally, as a physician and with equal passion, I resent having my patients turned into expense items.

Both you and I dislike the insurance companies and all the other fat cats at the top of the corporate food chain. We've voiced our opinions loud enough over the years that the government has stepped in and said they would help with various laws and regulations over the years, culminating recently in the Affordable Care Act. But is Washington only pretending to be our best friend and ultimate ally? Might the people in the beltway be something else entirely?

FIVE

Trust Betrayed

When things get out of control and we feel powerless to improve our lives, we have traditionally turned to the one entity we've come to consider our *ultimate* ally, the government. Since the creation of the United States of America, We The People have willingly delegated some of our power to the government. In return, the government is supposed to use the power we hand over for our benefit. This exchange has been increasingly abused over the years, but the idea still holds true.

Governments are made up of people we call public servants. Our City Councilman, State Senator, U.S. Congresspersons (Representatives and Senators), and certainly the President are all people we chose to serve us. They are supposed to make our lives better. If that isn't on the first line on their job descriptions, it should be.

Governments are created "by the people" for one purpose: to do those things for us that we cannot do for ourselves. We cannot defend ourselves from foreign aggression so the government creates and runs the military. We cannot build interstate highways, launch satellites for communication, or protect our natural resources, not as individuals. That is why we have federal, state, and municipal governments with their accompanying bureaucracies. Whether you think the government is doing well by us or not, the fact remains, that's what they are there for—to serve us, to care for us.

What about health care? When you become ill, can you take care of yourself? Occasionally yes, if it's the cold, a bout of the flu, or diarrhea. But what if it is more serious? What happens when you have acute appendicitis, a broken arm, or a heart attack? Does your next-door neighbor just happen to have an MRI scanner or a cardiac catheterization lab in his basement? Can your son whip up some antibiotics or possibly some Viagra® with his home chemistry set?

Obviously, the answer is "no." We need highly trained individuals and sophisticated technologies for our medical care. They are expensive, ... no, they are very expensive, ... okay, they are incredibly expensive. Ninety-nine percent of us cannot pay for all or even part of our medical bills, so we need help.

ACA isn't the first time that Washington has stepped in to protect us from "goliaths" of corporate greed whom we've always assumed are the multi-national insurance conglomerates. Our ultimate ally, the government, says it is there to create laws to protect us from big business making money off of us little guys, right?

Did you ever ask yourself, who or what is the most powerful and dangerous goliath?

Government Responses

Americans are fortunate to live in a country[1] where the federal government can't just shut a business down because it wants to or because the business doesn't support the party in power.[2] Governments can, however, create laws that control commercial activities, particularly healthcare, which is arguably the most highly regulated industry in the U.S.

Washington passes laws that are supposed to protect or help us. These Acts are merely words on paper that don't impact us until the rule-writing bureaucrats get involved. They interpret the laws and then write the rules and regulations that directly affect our day-to-day lives.

In terms of healthcare, various legislative acts have been passed presumably to control corporate greed. The intent behind such laws was ostensibly to ensure that everyone, especially our most vulnerable, would get their health needs met regardless of their financial condition.

As you will see later, asking Washington to protect us is literally asking cancer to cure cancer. Meanwhile, let's take a closer look at some healthcare laws—their purpose and their results—so we can see how effective the government has been at doing what they said they would do.

Medicare

Medicare is so much a part of our vocabulary that we have forgotten that it was once a bill that did not enjoy universal support (by a long shot.) Medicare was passed in 1965 to guarantee health care to people who had retired and therefore were theoretically no longer eligible for employer-supported health insurance. At that time, virtually all Americans got their health insurance where they worked. Thus, if you were no longer working, you were no longer able to get insurance. Medicare was the answer from our ultimate ally.

Medicare was set up as a government-run "Health Savings Account." It is very different from Medicaid, even though the two are sometimes confused. I will deal with Medicaid in a bit, but for now, know that Medic*aid* is a government entitlement program which means that if you qualify, you pay nothing for health care. Medic*are*, on the other hand, was supposed to be an old age medical savings account.

The idea wasn't a bad one: you paid in until you retired (you probably still do—it's listed right on your paystub), and then Medicare paid your health expenses afterward. Medicare was designed to use the Lockbox concept. You contributed money. The government put your cash in a small virtual lockbox with your name on it and then invested it at some modest but safe rate-of-return. With that money piling up over a forty-year working lifetime, growing at some nominal rate above inflation, there should be more than enough money for all your health care needs in the golden years.[3]

Now we hear that Medicare (like Social Security, another "lockbox" program gone bad) will run out of money between 2017 and 2027. If Medicare goes down, if it goes bankrupt, it won't "be there for us" when we need it. How did this happen? Where is your lockbox?

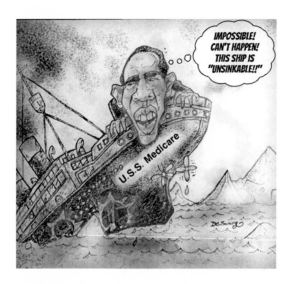

Sometime between 1965 and 1975, the cancer in the federal bureaucracy looked at all that nice, hard cash and thought, "I can't just let it sit there. I can do all sorts of things with cash, like spend it in ways that will make me bigger and more powerful." So, Congress *broke open* the lockbox, or should I say tens of millions of lockboxes. They took out all that cash, hundreds of billions of dollars, and put it into the General Account. There, they can use it for any purpose, any pet project, or to reward some crony capitalist of the party in power. The date this started is unknown because they never disclosed their pilferage to the public.

Technically, Congress had the legal right to use our money how it sees fit. According to the 1960 Supreme Court decision in Flemming v. Nestor, Congress can use money held in the U.S. Treasury acquired as tax revenue for any purpose it (Congress) deems proper.[4] So, they have the *legal* right to spend our money how they choose. Do they have the *moral* right?

Do you think it is okay for the government to take our hard-earned money, money that we diligently put away for health care needs in our later years, and use it for other things?

Congress has loudly assured us that they kept the books straight. They replaced our cash contributions with shiny, new government-issued I.O.U.s, claiming there was no difference.[5] Can you invest an I.O.U. like you can do with cash? That was a rhetorical question. Of course you can't. So how could your money or my money grow or even stay even with inflation? It couldn't, and it didn't.

That is how Congress created another massive unfunded liability. It broke its promise that we would receive whatever health care we needed after age sixty-five. You hear about it in the news all the time, "there is not enough money to pay for our old age medical care needs." No one ever says *why*—because our lawmakers, through their bureaucrats, raided our piggy banks called Medicare.

The government is made up of human beings; many of these people are good public servants, some not so much. Because Congress used our money elsewhere and cannot honor its health care commitments, someone—either a sinister lawmaker or a greedy bureaucrat, we'll never know for sure—came up with the "brilliant" idea to reduce payments to providers. They would make the books balance by simply paying the doctors less. (Are you surprised they never thought about paying the bureaucrats less?)

Multiple Directors of Medicare assured the American public that these reduced payments were only a "short-term" fix. This "short-term" fix has been continuing for thirty years, and the problem is now entirely out of control. Congress just recently passed another fix for Medicare called MACRA, the Medicare Access and Children's Health Insurance Reauthorization Act of 2015, which—surprise!—fixed nothing.[6]

The Medicare bureaucracy continues to assure us that it will cover all our old age health benefits, but will it really? More and more doctors cannot afford to accept Medicare payment schedules as the payments are below their cost-of-doing-business. What good is having Medicare coverage if it does not get you medical care?

I have a friend who manages a large Urology group practice (five doctors, nine nurses and seven staff). He reported a recent conversation that demonstrates what is happening.

One of the many new insurance carriers that have cropped up after passage of ACA called my friend, wanting to sign up his surgical group to provide services to the people they would enroll. The insurance manager asked if my friend's group was qualified and experienced in doing a certain procedure, let's call it operation "H." My friend said yes, two of their doctors did operation H often and had an excellent success rate.

"What will be the payment for doing that procedure," asked my friend?

Proudly and loudly, the insurance salesperson said, "Though we are a non-profit organization, we pay Medicare rates for operation H!" After a moment of silence, my friend asked, "Excuse me. Did you say Medicare rates, which for operation H is $1400?

"Yes, that is what I said," was the reply. "Did I mention that we are not-for-profit?"

My friend is not known for his (ahem) restraint. He screamed back the following. "Well, *you* may be not-for-profit, but we are in business. We need to take in more than we spend. The disposables alone for operation H cost us $1500. So that means every time we do the procedure, we will lose $100. Not to mention, I won't be able to pay my doctors or nurses. Are you crazy?!"

The rebuttal on the other end of the line was, just before my friend slammed down the phone, "But, but, we pay Medicare rates, and we are ... not-for-profit!"

Remember the old (unfunny) accounting joke that said, "Yes, it's true that I am losing money on each sale. But I'll make it up in volume!" The reason this isn't funny is because some people actually still believe that is possible. Apparently, this includes the members of Congress.

If you pay a businessperson—doctor, dry cleaner, dairy farmer—less than his or her expenses, they will go broke and have to go out of business.

The bottom line is this: us older citizens (over sixty-five) can't find a doctor to care for us because Medicare payments won't even cover the basic costs for procedures, let alone any kind of decent wages for the doctor. If you're thinking, "How is it right that the government, who is supposed to be our ally, promised us old age health care, and didn't deliver?" you are not alone.

Mean Well ≠ Do Well

Our allies—medical as well as governmental—loudly proclaim they mean well by us. Just look at the sign over every hospital front entrance in the country. It reads something like, "HERE, the patient comes first!" Reality can be ... otherwise. I wish the following weren't true, but I have seen it play out over and over in forty-one years of practicing medicine.

In healthcare, as in all activities, true priorities are often in conflict with publicly stated objectives. The bottom line is this: If finances are more important than patients, money will be "saved" by cutting our care services. If avoiding risk and being compliant with federal regulations are more important than what happens to us, then medical outcomes will not improve. It's classic double-speak, saying one thing but meaning another. After years of listening to this "speaking with forked tongue," I was able to compile this table. On the left hand side is what the public is told. The right-hand side is what it actually means:

Hospital Priorities		
Stated; Overt; Public	Priority	Actual; Unspoken; Covert
Quality patient care	1	Protect my position (Avoid CLA*)
Service to community	2	Service to the Board** or Oval Office
Research	3	Bottom line (financial)
Teaching	4	Compliance with regulations
	5	Avoid any and all risks
	6	Research or Teaching
	7	Perception in community
	8	Quality of patient care
	9	Service to patients
CLA*=career-limiting action. Board** refers to the Board of Directors, Regents, Trustees, or Supervisors, or Federal government, whoever is in charge.		

I hope you take the time to study this table so that you believe me when I write the following. Meaning well may turn into doing well for the provider—doctor, hospital, or insurance agent. Meaning well always turns out well for the politician and bureaucrat but almost never ends up good *for you* (the patient).

While there certainly are uncaring doctors, venal hospital CEOs, greedy insurance people, and grasping bureaucrats, I believe that most of these people actually *do* mean to do well. However, as I wrote earlier, what matters is not their intentions but our outcomes. In order to help you understand, let's take a look at the two government programs that could be considered the height of good intentions: Medicaid and EMTALA. As you read about them, ask yourself, "Has their meaning well actually *done well* for me?"

Medicaid

It feels right to provide health care for our less fortunate brethren. Medicaid was intended to do just that.

Medic*aid* became law the same year as Medic*are* (1965). To recap, Medicare is a system where people pay into the system and receive benefits in the future. Medicaid is different. It is like welfare. It's given for free to those in need and they get the benefits now.

Medicaid was originally constructed to provide health insurance for people who were *"unable to produce income,"* such as children, women during pregnancy, women with young children (at home), and the disabled. It has since become a means-tested program where the only qualifications are poverty and certain medical diseases. Ability or inability to generate income is no longer a factor.

Because Medicaid is a system that is supported by our tax dollars, it is the public's obligation to ask how well it has helped the less fortunate. The evidence unfortunately does not point toward success.

Coverage of poor Americans by Medicaid is spotty at best. Like Deamonte Driver's parents (the boy who died from complications of a cavity), twenty-four percent of those who are eligible for Medicaid's "free care" choose, for whatever reason, not to sign up. Maybe they know something we don't.

The hard data clearly shows that, at best, those with Medicaid insurance are no healthier than those with no insurance at all. At worst, having Medicaid coverage is associated with being sicker! Those statements are based on the following evidence, not on bias or personal opinion.

Katherine Baicker, PhD, of the Harvard School of Health Policy and Management, and her colleagues reported an experiment that was made possible by a partial expansion (under ACA) of the Medicaid program in the state of Oregon.[7] When they compared those who enrolled in Medicaid to those who stayed uninsured, they found that those with no insurance were just as healthy as those who had Medicaid insurance. In other words, having Medicaid insurance was no better for patients than having no insurance at all.

In different 2010 report, a different researcher named LaPar, found that Medicaid enrollees were actually sicker than those who had no insurance at all!

A big part of the problem is lack of doctors. The Medicaid reimbursement schedule is so low that it is below most doctors' cost of keeping their doors open. One third of U.S. doctors say they cannot see Medicaid patients because they cannot afford to.[8] The government reimbursement schedule is so low that the more Medicaid patients a doctor sees, the faster the doctor goes broke.

One has to wonder why our ultimate ally—the government—expanded the Medicaid program when it has such a poor track record of medical outcomes, and makes promises to deliver health care but has no doctors to see you.

EMTALA, Then UMRA

In the 1980s, the U.S. government observed a serious problem that was hurting many Americans: Many people had no health insurance and therefore no access to care. Sound familiar?

In earlier days, those who were ill but had no money could always fall back on their local county hospital. In Cook County, Illinois (Chicago's county), if you were ill, were poor and had no insurance, you could get the care you needed at Cook County Hospital, one of the largest and best municipal health care centers in the country.

In its heyday, Cook County had well over three thousand active beds to receive patients. Admittedly, some wards had as many as sixty patients in one big room. I remember those rooms well.

When I went to medical school (in the Pre-Cambrian era according to my son), every medical student in Chicago, regardless of which school you attended, got practical experience at Cook County Hospital. For Obstetrics and General Medicine, I trained at Cook County and received some of the best teaching a student could ever want.

People may say that I never had the opportunity to learn from a battlefield, like Korea or Viet Nam. Those individuals have never been in the Emergency Department of Cook County Hospital on a Saturday night. I have.

Cook County Hospital was a great institution. People got good care there, regardless of how little money they had. But, by the mid-1980s, that was no longer true in Chicago or anywhere else. Support for county hospital systems had dried up. Poor people who needed health care had no place to go.

In 1986, Congress passed EMTALA, the Emergency Medical Transport and Active Labor Act. With EMTALA as Law, a patient coming into an Emergency Department and needing acute care *must* receive care, by federal law. The hospital must provide it, even if patient has no money and no insurance, and regardless of how much that care will cost the hospital. Further, the hospital is forbidden to transfer that patient to another institution. Hence its nickname: the anti-dumping law.

EMTALA has helped millions of poor individuals who are here illegally. They are ineligible for government-supported insurance of any kind due to lack of legal citizenship. However, they are still eligible for unlimited "free" care under EMTALA.

That's great, but it's also open for massive waste, fraud, and abuse. If you can't go to a doctor's office because you don't have insurance, you can go to the emergency room. You can do that for anything from a hangnail to a heart attack. There are no restrictions, no checks and balances on the system.

EMTALA, though it fixed one problem, created a much bigger nightmare—the "unfunded mandate." Ever since 1986, U.S. hospitals are required by law to give care even if the hospital never gets paid. Such care is "free" to the patient. It is anything but free to the hospital and doctors who still have their own bills to pay.

Several years ago, while advising my own institution on how to avoid bankruptcy, I discovered ten patients who accounted for more than twelve million dollars a year of "free care." They were all in kidney failure and on dialysis. This was costing the hospital over $10,000 per patient per month. None of these patients had health insurance. The hospital had to absorb this yearly $12 million loss, by law.

To cope financially, hospitals have to "find" money elsewhere, or close their doors. There is no third alternative. Therefore, hospitals "over-charge" insured patients to make up losses mandated by EMTALA.

If you wonder why it costs you two dollars for an aspirin while in the hospital, that is because the hospital charges you extra so it can pay $10,000/month for a patient on dialysis who has no health insurance. You and I pay double for our health care: Once for ourselves and once again for the unfunded mandate.

With a seeming national scandal over hospitals gouging or over-charging insured patients (to make up for mandated losses), the federal government stood up, accepted responsibility, and said they would clean up their own mess. (I really wish they would have put it that way, but they didn't. They just created more useless legislation.)

In 1995, Congress passed UMRA, the Unfunded Mandates Reform Act. I won't bore you with the details, but you can see for yourself that UMRA did not reform anything: the problem of unfunded mandates remains unresolved. Hospitals are forced to over-charge us to stay in business. Though UMRA fixed nothing, it did accomplish one thing. It spent money, lots of it I suspect. Since Congress does not kept track of how much they spend on bureaucracy (on themselves), I cannot provide you with an exact number.

HIPAA—Totally Missing the Mark

Medicare, Medicaid, and EMTALA were at least trying to solve issues related to people's health care. The award for Congress' most misguided legislation before ACA—may I have the envelope, please—goes to HIPAA, The Health Insurance Portability and Accountability Act of 1996.

People outside the workings of healthcare know little or nothing about HIPAA. People inside healthcare turn their heads and spit when someone speaks its name.

The following is the problem that Congress said HIPAA would solve. During the economic turndown of the early 1990s, Americans were being laid off in droves. RIF (reduction in force: a military term) became the new euphemism for "getting your pink slip," that is, being fired from your job. When workers lost their jobs, they lost their employer-supported health insurance. Millions of previously insured Americans suddenly joined the ranks of the uninsured.

Our ultimate ally—Congress—promptly stepped in to rescue us. They began discussions of how to make health insurance "portable." Somewhere along the way, it was decided that confidentiality of medical information had to be protected at all costs, both literally and figuratively. The "P" (portability) part of the law, the reason that Congress became involved in the first place, gradually became lost or was forgotten.

HIPAA became the watchdog of medical informational security. Those who broke such security, i.e., failed to comply with HIPAA guidelines, had to be held *accountable*—the first "A" in HIPAA. Portability was never solved. People still lose their insurance when they lose their jobs.

Neither the public nor the providers get any benefit from HIPAA. What they do get are costs and shackles, respectively. While HIPAA expenses do not show up on any federal budget, you and I pay for it big time.

The ball and chain that HIPAA puts on providers is very real and hurts the public. You probably think that protecting our privacy is a good thing—and, of course, it is. But HIPAA is downright scary.[9]

Do you remember the uproar in the aftermath of the 9/11 tragedy, when we learned that the FBI, the CIA, and state and local law enforcement were not sharing information? Well, HIPAA makes it illegal for health providers to share information fully—and the consequences can be as devastating.

Suppose a psychiatrist puts you on a drug. Later, you go see your general doctor or you are in the Emergency Department with some other problem. The doctor who sees you will access your medical record, but guess what? He or she is not permitted to see what psychiatric drug(s) you are taking. HIPAA prevents that in the name of protecting confidentiality.

So, there is a good chance the second (current) doctor could put you on a drug that interacts badly with your psychiatric drug. The mix could harm, even kill, you. (Psychiatric medicines are by themselves very, very powerful, and suicide is a common side effect).

The reason this is happening is simple. The second doctor is not allowed to see the drugs the first doctor prescribed, by HIPAA law! Thank you, Congress. I worry that such errors happen thousands of times every year. Unfortunately, since no one is keeping track of any harm that might be done by Congressional legislation, I cannot provide a reliable number, and it would be irresponsible to guess.

As you can see, HIPAA is more than merely a waste of time for healthcare professionals. It is hazardous to your health. In George Orwell's novel *1984*, Big Brother was always there, everywhere.[10] Big Brother was Orwell's name for a governmental agency dedicated to watching you all the time—both your actions and even your thoughts. Those who didn't comply with government rules were re-educated (a "nice" way of saying punished).

To U.S. providers, HIPAA is Big Brother. He is watching us ... and frowning. We providers are not paranoid, not if they *are* out to get us! But with HIPAA, there is more, and it's worse.

HIPAA hides potentially unsafe regulations under something called "risk management." While everyone knows what the word risk means, most people do not know that hospital Departments of Risk

Management are not there to reduce medical risks *for patients*. They exist to prevent legal or financial risks *to the hospital*.

What is the big risk that every hospital Risk Management Department tries to reduce? It is being "out of compliance" with HIPAA guidelines.

HIPAA not only hurts the public medically and fails to protect the public from risk, but it costs us lots of money. You just can't count it.

HIPAA is a brilliant bureaucratic sleight-of-hand. The government avoids being seen as the policeman or the spendthrift (over-spending your money), even though it is both. How do they accomplish this neat trick? By turning the hospitals into policemen and spendthrifts. HIPAA requires hospitals to enforce a dizzying array of federal regulations. Worse, the hospitals must foot the bill for hundred of billions of dollars in costs to be in "regulatory compliance," costs that are necessarily passed on to you.

In each and every year for the past forty years (except the years 2000-2002), the national approval rating for the U.S. Congress has been below fifty percent. It has been below 30 percent for the past ten years. Can you imagine not just keeping but repeatedly *rewarding* your employees when more than two thirds of your customers think talking to your employees, in Congress' case *our* employee-Representatives, is a waste of time?

On Nov. 5, 2013, Congress achieved a new all-time low job approval rating of 8.8 percent! That means over ninety percent of Americans thought our Senators and Representatives were doing a bad job. Ever since the ACA was passed, Congress' job approval has stayed below twenty percent.[11] Looking at monstrosities like HIPAA or Obamacare, you can readily see why.

Government Guidelines: Nightmare of Compliance

Welcome to the *Brave New World* of government rules, regulations and guidelines.[12] While I delve into this subject in depth in chapter 7, I'm going to give you a peek into the horror show that these seemingly innocent "guidelines" create. This will help you understand how HIPAA and ACA became the nightmares they currently are.

Government regulations and guidelines claim they are simply there to help: to keep danger away and to make sure that doctors and nurses are providing the best care possible. Reality is far different.

First, it's important to understand what the government means by "guidelines."

The government uses a tried-and-true bureaucratic ploy called plausible deniability. Here's how it works. When asked about the high cost of HIPAA, your friendly government bureaucrat says, "We didn't make the hospitals or doctors do *anything*. We simply offer some ideas for them to consider. We just make some suggestions. We call them guidelines."

"Federal guidelines" is another example of doublespeak. They are in fact the very opposite of what you think they are. You might think that "guidelines" are suggestions or recommendations to help you when you make a choice. Not even close.

A friend and medical colleague—with the initials L.C.—wrote a book several years ago titled *A Guide to Biking in New Mexico.*" L.C.'s book has *real* guidelines. It shows you various routes to take. You decide where you want to go. It discusses the degrees of difficulty on each route. You choose how hard a ride you want. The guidebook warns you which route has more thorn bushes. You decide whether you want to use (heavier) thorn-resistant tires and put a sealant called Slime® inside the tubes. The guidelines give you options and alternatives. You use your best judgment. You decide.

If the Federal government were writing the same biking guidebook, it would dictate the kind of bike you must ride, the precise time to leave, the speed you must use on each leg of the journey, and of course, the destination. If you rode according to "federal guidelines," you would have no choices at all.

Most of us have stolen something at some time—from a kiss to a candy bar to someone else's idea. We're never proud of it, but it happens. Infractions happen all the time. If we're lucky, we get caught. We made amends, and we learn.[13] Life moves on.

There is more flexibility in a steel rod than in government guidelines. You follow them to the letter, *or else*. And that is no idle threat.

The useless (but expensive) piece of legislation titled HIPAA affects everyone and everything having to do with healthcare. And if that's not bad enough, here's where it gets scary, insane, or both. After Congress passed HIPAA, hospital lawyers around the country reviewed the guidelines very carefully. They found the most extreme interpretations and then made hospital employees toe that line. This includes all health-care workers, from doctors and nurses, to respiratory therapists and maintenance or support staff.

For example: HIPAA says nothing about whether the Internet is considered secure or not. However, highly risk-averse hospital lawyers forbid your doctor from communicating with outside doctors by email—the very doctors who may have vital information about your health and information needed to make an accurate diagnosis.

Another example: HIPAA created a whole series of learning modules about medical information security and other arcane subjects in healthcare. It then "suggested" that healthcare workers study these modules. If you wonder why your doctor has less than five minutes to see your child, it is because she or he has to spend hours in front of a computer studying HIPAA security compliance modules, take tests on this useless information, and then have the proper hospital officials sign off on proof of the doctor's compliance. I know because I took hundreds of those tests. If I didn't, the hospital wouldn't have allowed me to practice medicine there.

Yet another example: HIPAA "suggested" that tighter security measures should be imposed on all venues with medical information, such as computers, doctors' notes, hospital charts, consultation letters, lab results, and procedure reports. Under HIPAA "guidelines," a patient's name must not be visible on the hospital chart. That means that the doctor, while still trying like hell to be efficient, has to guess which chart is yours. How many errors have resulted from writing wrong notes or incorrect orders in a chart? I know it happens. I have done it.

Here's the kicker on the "guideline" scam: the government doesn't pay for all that increased security activity and built-in inefficiency. I can envision some politician shouting into a microphone, "And, voting public, there is no charge for all our sage advice that protects you from those negligent doctors. It costs you absolutely nothing. You don't have to pay us a cent!"

While it might not show up on your tax bill, you do pay for it, and through the nose. The bills are indirect, sent via the hospitals, professional societies, insurance companies, drug companies, licensing bureaus, etc. Regardless of who sends the actual bill, the government made such spending a legislative requirement, *or else*! You and I have to pay it.

If you think I'm joking, take a look at the computer screens in your doctor's office, the dentist's office, or in the hospital. They are all fitted with polarizing screens so that a passer-by cannot see what is on the computer screen. Not necessarily a bad idea but is it worth the hundreds of millions of dollars required to retrofit every medical computer in the U.S.? I doubt it, especially since the public ends up paying for them. But since we bear these costs *indirectly*, the government can pretend that the expenses don't exist.

Penalties for Non-Compliance

The government has learned that "guidelines" give them a mighty big club, and they're not afraid to wave it around, even use it. There are also spikes on the end of the club—stiff penalties levied against those who do not follow government rules to the letter. Both hospitals and doctors are routinely threatened with "Regulatory Review." If you're found to be non-compliant, then the doctor can lose her right to practice medicine or the hospital can lose its license. Both are then out of business.

So hospitals and doctors work like hell to make sure they're "In Compliance." The costs are astronomical, both in dollars and in lives compromised or lost altogether. "Regulatory Review" is how Congress gets medical institutions to do its bidding, *and to pay for it*. Of course, you know who pays in the end, you do.

I've mentioned this before, but it bears repeating because it's so insidious. HIPAA is one of the many costly burdens of regulatory compliance that never show up on any budget sheet. It is an expense item that probably runs into the hundreds of billions. Yes, I wrote billions with a "b." That's a hell of a lot more than all the money lost through fraud and abuse.

How much does regulatory compliance cost, exactly? No one knows. The costs for HIPAA as one example, both direct and indirect, are unknown. They are quite intentionally hidden, buried in the expenses of *necessary* bureaucracy.

Regulatory compliance is a huge, invisible sinkhole. No, worse, it is a black hole.[14] It sucks in healthcare dollars, increasing our insurance premiums and our copayments—the part of the hospital bill that our insurance doesn't cover. Regulatory compliance makes your service worse, not better. Doctors and nurses are so busy making sure they are HIPAA compliant, they have very little time for you, the patient.

How is it right that the government, the entity that is supposed to be our ultimate ally, puts a stumbling block like HIPAA directly in front of the nurses and doctors who are simply trying to care for their patients? Having lived under the weight of federal guidelines for over forty years at several different hospitals, I can say with certainty that the writers of federal healthcare guidelines are not concerned about your health or welfare.

HIPAA and other Acts demonstrate the government's real intent: To enlarge the bureaucracy. Compliance oversight is an important tool to help the bureaucracy grow. The hospitals and people who provide your care are "rewarded" by having punishment withheld. There is no carrot, only a stick for the non-compliant and a bonus for the compliance officer.

ACA—Latest, Not Greatest

All of our government's previous attempts to fix our ailing healthcare system—from Medicare and Medicaid to EMTALA and HIPAA—have produced the mess President Obama inherited in 2008.

Wasting no time after taking office, Mr. Obama made solving healthcare's dysfunction his top, indeed his only, priority. He pointed to a growth rate in healthcare spending our nation couldn't afford. He highlighted health care that individual Americans couldn't afford, and he called the tens of millions of uninsured Americans a "stain on our national honor."

While he "didn't build that" [the U.S. healthcare system], he promised that he could fix it. The President immediately latched on to the British model of government-controlled healthcare. He decided to emulate its vaunted National Health Service (NHS) as the solution for the U.S.

I have considerable personal experience with the NHS. Before college, I went to school in England but that was a long time ago. More recently, my son went to graduate school in London. When he became ill, he did not qualify for care through the NHS because he wasn't a British citizen. And then the NHS tried to kill my mum.

I was blessed with two mothers. My biological mother was American (mom). My adoptive mother was British (mum). My mom in New York paid large sums every month for both health insurance and co-payments. She lived to age ninety-six and one-half years, never in a nursing home, and was sharper than the rest of us for ninety-six and a quarter of those years.

My English mum had free health care through the NHS and their so-called universal health care system. (It wasn't "universal" for my son.) Mum was a midwife in northwestern England. Shortly before her eightieth birthday, she slipped and broke her hip. She could no longer work or even walk, and thus was confined to bed. Her doctor said she needed a hip replacement. Fortunately, under the British system, it would be free. On a midwife's salary, mum did not have the money to pay for major surgery.

Her doctor asked for and received authorization from the NHS for mum's hip replacement. He immediately called her with the good news. She smiled and asked him when she would have surgery. Her three sons wanted to know too. Only then did the doctor pay attention to the Date of Operation on the approval form. Mum was in the queue—British word for line—to have her surgery two years and three months in the future.

You do not have to be a physician to know this was a death sentence. Putting a seventy-eight-year old over-weight woman at strict bed rest makes her completely immobile. She would certainly become more obese, probably develop pneumonia, a stroke, or a pulmonary embolus (blood clot in the lungs).

Obviously, she could no longer work and be productive, or even live at home. She would need to be in a nursing home with all the attendant costs. She would likely die before her scheduled surgery, thus avoiding the expense of her operation.

The government that was supposed give my mum the medical care she needed, instead gave her a number to stand (or in her case lie in bed) in line so she could die waiting for the surgery. Mum's ultimate ally, the government healthcare system, sentenced her to death by inaction.

This was the model that President Obama chose to solve the problems of U.S. healthcare. In chapter 10, we will evaluate all the facts of what Obamacare, the ACA, has done *to* us (sadly not *for* us.) Here, I want to point out that the approach chosen by the President—the NHS—could not deliver what he promised us it would.

I did not write wouldn't. I wrote *couldn't*.

There is solid evidence how the British system functions.[15] Its actions would be anathema to Americans if we only knew about them. The President's model for healthcare in America, the NHS: (a) excludes non-citizens from government care, and (b) uses strict medical rationing to control costs.[16] I bet you did not know that rationing is a critical element in the ACA. Mr. Obama neglected to mention that to us.

With rationing, you get what medical care the government allows your doctor to use, not "all the care that Americans deserve," and most definitely not the care you need to stay alive. If you are over fifty-five years old and need kidney dialysis, under the British system, you won't get it. You just die. ACA's Independent Payment Advisory Board (IPAB) is a duplicate of the NHS. So presumably, IPAB and the ACA will cut costs the same way, by medical rationing.

Medical rationing, no doctors to see us, money disappearing, insurance we can't afford, care we can't possibly pay for, allies becoming enemies—while the insurance companies have definitely lined their pockets with our money, the government, with its continual promise to help, has betrayed us with every "fix" it puts forth as law. It hurts very badly when trust is betrayed, just like cancer causes pain, often severe.

In the introduction, we exposed the cancer of uncontrolled greed and unrestrained power in our healthcare system. In chapter 2 and this chapter we got upset as we learned how much of our money Washington is taking and spending on healthcare. If trillions of dollars are pouring into government coffers, why can't Americans get the health care (two words) we need?

SIX

The Root Cause

Recently, I waited in line for twenty minutes at the post office. It was around 11:30, lunchtime. There was one clerk. The other one was at lunch and came back to his post right before it was my turn. I know my post office clerks fairly well, so I remarked that the guy who used to work down at the end of the counter must have retired because he hadn't been there in a while. My clerk told me that he actually got transferred to a post office closer to his home.

I then asked, "What about the gal who used to work right next to you?"

He said that she got promoted, that another coworker was still on vacation, and, "They're not going to replace the guy who got transferred."

I said, "Really? Even with lines this long?"

The clerk said matter of factly, "They're trying to get this office down to just one of us."

I deadpanned, "You're kidding."

He said, "No, it's good for business. It reduces our costs. If people are willing to wait in line, then why not?"

I thanked him for helping me, then I left, shaking my head. The post office just raised its prices on everything except the stamp. They also now close their doors at 5:00 or 5:30 p.m. If you work until 5 and you're too far away to get the post office, too bad.

As I walked to my car, I thought, "No, making people wait far too long to mail a package is not good for business. It's good for the bureaucracy."

Think about this: The post office is cutting service—fewer clerks, shorter hours. But they are taking *more* of our money—their prices have just gone up. In other words, the post office is taking our money while cutting our service.

The healthcare system is far more complex than the post office, but the premise still holds. The system is taking our money but cutting our service.

In the introduction, I wrote that the healthcare bureaucracy was acting like a cancer. It is growing, expanding greedily out of control because the bureaucracy—not the actual care patients receive—costs so much money.

The post office worker annoyed me, but more importantly, he validated what I have known for years. The "system" is the bureaucracy. The health care bureaucracy, like any federal, state, or local government bureaucracy, *takes our money and cuts our service.* Federal healthcare bureaucrats serve the cancer, not us, and the cancer is driving the bureaucracy to seek unrestrained power and uncontrolled greed. Because the healthcare bureaucracy has this pernicious type of cancer, it will continue to take our money and cut our service. It is a dwindling spiral. The prognosis is not good, maybe even grim.

Can Bureaucracies Be Greedy?

I have talked at length about how much money the government is spending on our healthcare system. The various laws reputedly passed to fix problems in healthcare have only made things more difficult for us. The Affordable Care Act is the worst. It takes more and more of our hard-earned money, and makes it harder to find a doctor. Put simply, Obamacare drastically *reduces* our ability to receive or to pay for medical care. We got the precise opposite of what was promised.

People are pointing fingers, but very few are actually calling out the real culprit, the entity that has grown like a monster, its ugly maw wide open, waiting to devour more of our money. They haven't taken action because they don't recognize that government bureaucracy is the problem.

I recently asked my good friend and physician colleague Paul what came to mind when he read the phrase "greedy bureaucracy." He answered, "I don't think of these words greed and bureaucracy together. My immediate thought of bureaucracy is government, at any level. But I don't think most government bureaucrats are greedy. Some are, but I really do think that most of them think they are doing the right thing (of course, they seldom actually accomplish the right thing, but that's a horse of a different color)."

Because bureaucrats are people just like you and me, my friend believed that they weren't all *that* greedy. He did concede that bureaucrats don't make anything we buy or do anything that directly helps us, the way a nurse, a policeperson, or a plumber does. Bureaucrats are actuaries, auditors, rule-makers, interpreters (lawyers), IRS agents, compliance officers, and the like. Paul works in a hospital and has been subject to all the same rules and regulations that I have, but he didn't equate that with greed. In fact, he insisted that the word greed was always associated with capitalism. He said that commerce is greedy but government and bureaucracy are not.

That is exactly what the bureaucracy wants you to believe. It's someone or something else that's causing all the problems. But if all the other problem areas have been hog-tied through legislation, and the problem still hasn't been solved, then it is time to shine the bright light of truth on what the cancer-ridden healthcare bureaucracy does:

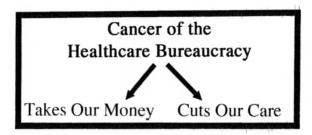

What Is Bureaucracy?

Bureaucracy is one of those words we all use but few understand. Think about it. Can you define it? Do you know why it began in the first place?

Bureaucracy can be defined as "government administration managed by departments staffed with nonelected officials." In modern times, bureaucracy refers to the administrative system that controls any large organization, institution, or a country.

All systems need some amount of organization, administration, and bureaucracy.

Historians argue over when bureaucracy started. Some say it began as far back as 4,000 B.C. with the Sumerians. Others say that Confucius invented bureaucracy in Ancient China around 450 B.C. It was something that governments need to administer other work. Confucius specifically intended bureaucracy to keep the government free from corruption. (What do you think he would say if he saw what his invention has become?)

In America, government bureaucracies include the agencies and offices that run Medicare, Welfare, the Department of Energy, National Institutes of Health, the Federal Food and Drug Administration (a.k.a. the FDA), the Department of Education, as well as thousands of others.

Somewhere along the way, the federal bureaucracy lost its true purpose. The following story is made up but it illustrates exactly what happens over and again in the world of government bureaucracy:

> Once upon a time there was a vast scrap yard in the middle of a desert, owned by the federal government.
> No one knew what was there or whether it was valuable.

In a subcommittee meeting, someone asked if it was possible for a thief to steal from the scrap yard at night. So, Congress created a night watchman position (GS-4) and hired a person for the job, then a second person to cover when the first was on vacation.

"How does the watchman do his job without an instruction manual," asked a Senate subcommittee? So they created a planning position and hired two people: one person to write the instructions (GS-12) and one person to do time studies (GS-11).

Then Congress said, "How will we know the night watchman is doing the tasks correctly?" Therefore, they created an Oversight Agency, starting with two people, one GS-09 to do the studies and one GS-11 to write the reports. This soon escalated to an entire organizational chart with boxes (and people) reporting to other boxes (and people) all with GS ratings of 09 to 12.

Then Congress said, "How are these people going to get paid?" So they created a Department within the Government Accounting Office, starting with a timekeeper (GS-09) and a payroll officer (GS-11). Within a year, there were eleven employees, GS-08 to GS-12.

Congress worried, "Who will be accountable for all of these people?" So they created an Agency Directorship (GS-16), who then hired three additional people: an Admin. Officer (GM-13); an Assistant Admin. Officer (GS-13); and a Legal Secretary (GS-08).

Later, the Agency Director testified before Congress that, "We have had this command in operation for one year and are now $18,000 over budget, we must cutback on costs."

So, they laid off both night watchmen. The bureaucrats lived happily ever after with their jobs, their benefits, and their pensions.

How can one explain this behavior, this series of events? Somewhere, somehow, the bureaucrats lost their focus, forgot their purpose, and changed bureaucracy's *raison d'être*.

Bureaucracy's *Raison D'être*

Raison d'être is French for reason-to-be, meaning the purpose for existence of someone or something. A crankshaft is in your car to transfer the power of the engine to the wheels. Its *raison d'être* is to make the car go.

All healthcare systems everywhere have the same, single *raison d'être*: to improve and protect the health of the people. Just as a car has various parts like engine, wheels, headlights, and seats, so a healthcare system has "parts" called providers, hospitals, insurance, and bureaucracy or you can call it administration and regulation.

Bureaucracy is a necessary part of any company, agency or government. The *raison d'être* for bureaucracy is straightforward: it helps all the other parts do their jobs. It has no job of its own other than being a lubricant and central switchboard.

Bureaucracy in a business helps the Sales Department sell; makes sure the Service Department services; and facilitates the Billing Department as it collects money. In the military, the bureaucracy assures that the Army knows what the Navy is doing and makes *sure* the soldiers have what they need to defend themselves—where, when, and how much is required whether it is armor, bullets, radios, or food.

What happened in the scrapyard? What altered bureaucracy's purpose? It developed cancer.

What Is Cancer?

I have already explained how cancer in a human body works. To help you understand how deeply dangerous the cancer of unrestrained greed and uncontrolled power is, I'm going to use another analogy. Cancer is like a nasty virus. It invades a cell in your body or a system like healthcare, and changes its *raison d'être*. Cancer is an evil reprogrammer.

When cancer invades your kidney, it tells the organ to stop filtering your blood and to start growing. When cancer takes control of a bureaucracy, it tells the bureaucrats to stop helping others, grab all the money they can, and spread out.

Regardless of the type of cancer or where it takes hold, cancer forces its host to do one thing and one thing only: GROW.

In this way, cancer is like Ebola or Hanta. These are viruses that invade parts of your body that you need to live. When the virus invades certain critical parts of your body, it reprograms the cells to stop doing their vital functions and just multiply. Ebola stops your coagulation system so you bleed to death internally. Hanta prevents your lungs from working so you die from lack of oxygen.

Cancer is the master reprogrammer. Whether the cancer is in your body or in our healthcare system, either way, it reprograms for growth, stops vital functions, and we die.

The Root Cause

Healthcare's primary problem is not insurance companies making obscene profits; they are simply playing the game the way Washington set up the rules. Nor is it the massive chasm between Democrats and Republicans, as some would like to believe. Both political parties have done their fair share of expanding government bureaucracy and thus encouraging the spread of this cancer. Some have even called the federal bureaucracy the "fourth branch of government," claiming that the bureaucracy is the *real* government.[1]

When a cancer of greed and power, with its ability to re-purpose, invades a bureaucracy that is susceptible to cancer because it has nothing to restrain it, you have a recipe for disaster. We are experiencing that disaster, the root cause, on a daily basis.

A *cancer of unrestrained greed and uncontrolled power within a government bureaucracy is the root cause for progressive deterioration of the American healthcare system.*

No Free-Market Restraint

Most people believe that, absent a miracle of modern medicine, cancer is a death sentence. Accepted wisdom says when you get it, that's it.

In fact, cancer can only thrive when the environment is friendly to it, i.e., where natural protective mechanisms are absent or suppressed.

The intestines in your body make millions of new cells every day to replace the old ones that live for less than 24 hours. At least 99.99 percent of the new cells you create are healthy and cancer-free, but a few will have cancer.

If your immune system is intact,[2] it will immediately recognize the cancer cells as being malignant. Immune cells or "protector cells" will destroy the new cancer cells before they can grow. This is happening every minute of every day inside your body.

Government bureaucracy doesn't have an immune system, obviously. Interestingly, the for-profit world of commerce does. Free market forces act like the immune cells in your body. They prevent the unrestrained growth of cancer. The commercial world has protection (free market forces) against cancer's growth: the world of government doesn't.

"Free market forces" refers to what happens when **supply** (of anything) and **demand** (for the same thing) are balanced by the individual decisions of millions of consumers spending their own money. The consumer chooses what to buy and the sellers compete for consumer dollars.

In a free market, a business that spends too much on its administrative bureaucracy will have to sell its product at too high a price. When consumers won't buy the over-priced product, the overspending business will soon be gone. In a free market, the danger of bankruptcy is a powerful incentive to spend less … or else.

Consumers in a free market have the same concern—bankruptcy—that sellers have. The consumer takes his money out of his wallet to buy. The consumer cannot spend more than he has or, like the overspending company, he will find himself in bankruptcy court.

In the commercial world, a cancer that tries to spend and grow without limit will soon be stopped by the restraining effect of free market forces.

A government does not have to pay attention to free market forces. It has no fear of bankruptcy. They can always print more money. There is no incentive within the government structure to save money. The government has no constraint or "brake" on its spending. There is nothing to prevent the cancer's unlimited expansion. Government bureaucracies like the EPA, FDA and Obamacare simply spend as much as they can get their hands on, diverting whatever money they can find to the cancer. Government bureaucracies have no reason to economize and so ... they don't.

Bureaucratic Diversion

Once you understand that it's the *bureaucracy* that is growing out of control, then you can start to see its effects everywhere. Just above, I used a simple, seemingly innocuous word, divert. In fact, *diversion* of funds is one of the most devastating tools a cancerous bureaucracy uses. It happens in all activities that government controls, not just healthcare but also infrastructure, the military, social services like food stamps—you get the idea.

Say an old bridge over a river is unstable. We need a new one. The government allocates a certain amount of money to build the new structure. Then the bureaucrats get to work deciding how much money goes to what. They determine how many forms in triplicate are needed; how many safety inspectors and compliance officers (same thing); and the number of directors, managers, and union liaison positions. What is left is used for I-beams, cables, and steel workers' salaries. The bureaucracy has *diverted* money to itself that should be used to build the bridge.

In Iraq, why did our military personnel carriers lack proper armor?[3] It's not because the colonels and generals were personally getting rich like insurance CEOs. The cancer in government bureaucracy made everything complex and convoluted, which means expensive. Money spent on bureaucrats—managers, inspectors, and lawyers—left less money for the troops. Bureaucratic diversion puts our soldiers' lives in jeopardy.

When there is bureaucratic diversion in healthcare, the life in jeopardy is yours.

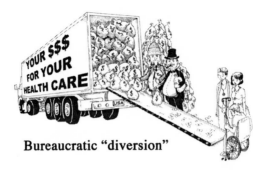

Bureaucratic "diversion"

Say a truck arrives with the money to pay for your health care. It is filled to the top with moneybags—$2.6 trillion dollars. That is the amount of your money that the government will spend on Obamacare.[4] Down comes the ramp and the moneybags start rolling out.

Standing closest to the truck opening is the government bureaucrat. He (or she) gets first crack at the money. The huge pile of your money behind him represents what he thinks he can get away with. He will spend it all and even more, claiming he is doing it for your own good.

Next to him is the corporate executive. His pile of moneybags is much smaller. He took only the amount he needed to make the maximum profit allowed by law. If he spends too much, he will make no profit and go broke.

Standing at the bottom of the ramp are patients, doctors and nurses. They (we) get the leftovers after bureaucrats take the lion's share.

We are talking about huge sums of money. These are *healthcare* dollars that produce no health … *care*.

When researchers at Harvard studied "The Cost of Healthcare Administration,"[5] they found that 31 percent of U.S. healthcare dollars went to government bureaucracy, administration, rules, regulation, and compliance—what I have named BARRC (The next chapter explains BARRC in greater depth.) My own analysis of the federal budget suggests the amount is even higher: 40 percent. Either way, we are talking about over *one trillion "inefficient" healthcare dollars.*

Dollar efficiency is defined as the percent of dollars going into a company or a system that produces the desired output or outcome. In an auto manufacturing plant, dollar efficiency is the number of dollars that result in a car to sell. You can be sure that Ford and Honda know their dollar efficiency down to the penny.

The same thing is true for the American Heart Association, the Red Cross, and Salvation Army. In a charitable organization, management is required by law to calculate and report how many of the dollars donated actually provide food, shelter, or supported training and research.

Every commercial activity, whether for-profit or not-for-profit, must measure and report its dollar efficiency to the federal government. That is the law.

The federal government makes the laws, yet there is no law that requires government bureaucracy to measure its own dollar efficiency. So the bureaucracy doesn't. Thus, bureaucrats can then say with a straight face, "We don't know." That is how they hide vital information from the public. Search on Google to find out how much government bureaucracy costs. The figures don't exist. However, you can easily download an annual report on any insurance company on the Internet that shows exactly how much the company spent.

We know trillions of dollars are diverted to government bureaucracy because the money that goes into the system does not equal the money being spent for services. This begs the very obvious question: what does the government bureaucracy do with all that money? Some goes to line the pockets of existing bureaucrats. Check out "bureaucrat salaries" on any Internet search engine. You will find information like "the growth of six-figure salaries [in federal bureaucracies] has pushed the average federal worker's pay to $71,206 compared with $40,331 in the private sector."[6]

The bulk of bureaucratically diverted money goes to cancer's growth. The government hires new bureaucrats with a multitude of names: actuary, accountant, biller, coder, compliance officer, consultant (does the name Jonathan Gruber ring a bell?), etc. Then, there are all the new physical facilities from buildings and roads to furniture, electricity, and computers ... and liability insurance. Don't forget all the lawyers needed to interpret and re-interpret the newly created rules, regulations and Acts. They will of course have to defend the bureaucrats when their rulings are challenged.[7]

Keep in mind that you and I pay for all this bureaucracy, from bureaucrats' paychecks and pension plans, to the super-expensive, use-government-approved-only printers in their offices. When I write, "they take our money and cut our care," the politicians are diverting money from medical care we need to enlarge a bureaucracy that we don't need.

Here is an example of bureaucratic diversion from my own personal experience as the Consumer Advocate member of the Board of Directors of our State-based Health Insurance Exchange. It is implementing the ACA. In this role, I am a bureaucrat (not a role that I or any doctor enjoys.)

When our Board calculated the cost of Information Technology (IT) services, the first estimate was just over $25 million. Why so much, especially for one of the least populous states in the Union? Because of the volume of bureaucratic data that Washington says we must acquire, manipulate, secure, and store. After we started to build the system they demanded, Washington kept altering the system design. Those change-orders increased the cost to over $50 million. That was just for IT.

Now, add the costs of outreach, education, marketing, internal bureaucracy, not to mention my magnificent salary (zero). We will spend over $100 million dollars, which makes those dollars *unavailable for patient care.*

Healthcare.gov is the federally created website for ACA-insurance in those twenty-one states that decided not to build state-based Insurance Exchanges. Do you know how much healthcare.gov cost? Take a guess. I bet you will be wrong by a factor of a thousand.

If you know anything about building a website you know that a million dollars would be a lot of money to build one. What would you say to the government spending over $2 billion, with a "b" for a website?![8] One that only works some of the time for us, but is wide open to hackers?

For a moment, let me take off my bureaucrat hat and put on my doctor cap. This expenditure makes me nauseous. For what the federal bureaucracy spent on a website, pediatric cardiologists like me could fix every child with a heart problem in the entire U.S., maybe the world! Wouldn't the money be better spent on our children than on an unnecessary and unreliable website?

The bureaucracy obviously doesn't think so. When you realize the healthcare bureaucracy would rather pay itself billions than give us the care we need, you know you are facing a cancerous bureaucracy.

Complexity As A Weapon

Perhaps the most powerful weapon in cancer's arsenal is complexity. Most people believe that modern life is naturally complex. Something as huge as a healthcare system is bound to be complex; thus people accept complexity as inevitable and unavoidable. That is just what the cancer wants you to do.

Inherent Complexity

One look at natural complexity will quickly show you how different it is from artificial or intentional complexity. The human body is extremely complex, by its very nature. Tens of thousands of different processes are going on in various organs, all at the same time. Yet—and here's the best part—by design, it is simple to use!

You are probably reading this book sitting down. Over time, you may become stiff. So you stand up to stretch your back. You don't consciously take stock of which muscles you must relax and which ones you have to contract. You don't look down to check where the floor is, or where your legs are in relation to your arms. You pay no attention to what your liver is doing to produce the energy that your muscles need. You don't care how much blood must be diverted from your stomach to your legs. You just … stand up. It's a complex system built to be remarkably simple for the end-user: You.

Another example of an inherently-complex-yet-simple-to-use design is my Apple laptop computer. It's what I'm using right now to write this down. To do that, I use the latest word processing program. To verify my facts, I access the Internet through a web browser on the same computer. To generate the tables of data, I use a spreadsheet program. To create graphics, I use two other programs.

Programs like Microsoft Word, Adobe Acrobat, Firefox web browser, Microsoft Excel, and Adobe Photoshop are incredibly complex. Yet someone like me, who knows nothing about programming, can operate them because they were built to be simple to use.

Management wisdom teaches that "nuclear submarines are designed by geniuses to be run by dummies." While the seamen who crew our submarines are anything but stupid, the aphorism makes an important point. When you design something complex like a submarine, a computer, an organization, or a large system like healthcare, the better you design it, the less complex it is for the end-users.

Simplicity is the hallmark of a brilliant—engineers call it elegant—design. What does it say about healthcare that it is convoluted, redundant, impenetrable, contradictory, and virtually incomprehensible to the system's end-users: Patients and doctors?

Artificial or Intentional Complexity

By the word artificial, I mean unnatural, not inherent as complexity is in your body. Artificial complexity is introduced intentionally into a system where it is not naturally present. Health care need not be so complex. It is that way because cancer wants it to be that way.

In a free market, if a product or service is too complex to use, consumers just don't buy it. We shop around until we find something that is easy to use, and we buy that. Competition in a free market forces producers to sell what consumers want. We want things that are easy, not complex. If sellers don't offer simple-to-use things for sale, they die… commercially, not literally.

Our healthcare system is the opposite of user-friendly. It's so complex that the system is virtually incomprehensible to everyone. I have an MD and an MBA and have been inside the healthcare system for over forty years. I don't fully understand it. Anyone who says he does is delusional or is lying to you.

Healthcare was designed to be incomprehensible *intentionally*. Complexity serves the purpose of a bureaucracy controlled by cancer—to get bigger, and Bigger, and BIGGER.

The competition that benefits consumers in a free market doesn't exist in government bureaucracy. We HAVE to buy what the government is selling and at the price they say. It's the (ACA) law. Sellers like insurance companies must sell what the government says they must sell. They can't compete to sell what the consumers want. We have no alternative to ACA-compliant insurance. Anything else is illegal.

You cannot say we weren't warned. U.S. President (1809-1817) James Madison sagely wrote, "In framing a government which is to be administered by men over men, the great difficulty lies in this: You must first enable the government to control the governed; and in the next place oblige it to control itself."[9]

President Madison never envisioned what we have now: A government that has been taken over by cancer, which keeps magnifying administrative complexity.

Before I retired, my hospital bought a new, expensive computer system for *e-prescribing*, writing medication orders for patients electronically. This replaced the old method of writing (often illegibly) on a prescription pad and giving the hand-written prescription to the patient. Sounds like a good idea, right?

In theory, a computer system offers huge advantages such as reducing errors, improved speed and efficiency, and automatically integrating medication orders with the electronic medical record. Electronic prescribing in fact does none of those things.

Rather than being simple for the end-user/doctor, e-prescribing is much harder; more expensive; takes longer; and introduces errors, all because of its artificial complexity.

In the old days (five years ago), I used to write on a piece of paper: "Penicillin, 250mg tabs; Take one every twelve hours by mouth, Dispense 20, No Refills." This took about thirty seconds. I would hand the paper to the patient and make sure he or she knew what it was, why they were taking it, and what to expect, including possible side effects.

With the new, complex e-prescribing system, I now have to login to three different systems using only government-approved computers, and then go through at least twenty-five different selections on various screens. Some of these screens have fifty or more choices from which to select. Next, I have to wait while the computer refreshes the electronic record and then validates what is on the new screen. Then the e-prescription could finally be printed out but only on a hyper-expensive government-approved printer. This entire process takes anywhere from ten to twenty-five minutes, assuming one of the systems hasn't crashed.

According to benchmark efficiency standards, I am supposed to see one Established Patient (one I have seen before) every fifteen minutes. If

I must use all that time just to write a prescription, how am I supposed to know what to write?! I have no time to talk with you, do a physical exam, look at test results, or think!

Obamacare offers a host of great examples of intentional, artificial complexity. I will restrain myself and simply give you two.

One easy measure of complexity could be the number of words. There are 8061 words in the Constitution of the United States including all twenty-seven ratified Amendments. The first round of regulations for the ACA—an insurance and tax bill—contains 10,516,000 words.[10] Lawyers have a Latin phrase that applies nicely: *res ipsa loquitur*, the thing speaks for itself.

Government forms are a second example of artificial bureaucratic complexity. We've all filled them out, or tried to. Nobody understands them. They are too complex. For instance, one question out of the 145 questions on a new ACA insurance forms asks: "Does your employer offer a health plan that meets the minimum value standard*?"

The asterisk *clarifies* for you how to answer the question. I cite directly from an ACA application form. "(*)=An employer-sponsored health plan meets the 'minimum value standard' if the plan's share of the total allowed benefit costs covered by the plan is no less than 60 percent of such costs (Section 36B(c)(2)(C)(ii) of the Internal Revenue Code of 1986)."[11] This is what they call *clarification*?! Of course not. It is intended to be so complex that the bureaucracy can justify spending more money on people to help translate what all that gobbledy-gook means.

Here comes the "navigator."

Your Savior—The Navigator

Federal bureaucrats who wrote the ACA created an impenetrable fog of rules, regulations, revisions, advisories, etc. You cannot see where you are going or what they are doing. You can't breath. You are lost, confused, and frightened, terrified that you won't be able to comply with federal mandates.

This fog of words created intentionally by government keeps expanding and thickening, with more and more (and more and more) words, like those shown below.

A Fog Of Government Rules You Are Expected to Obey
• If you fail to submit Form 1098A before April 15, the penalty …
• The procedure requested for you by your doctor is not authorized.
• Form 1098A has been changed to 1098C. You must re-file no later than...
• Section 103, paragraph 11 requires you to …
• The PCIP Program has been temporarily suspended.
• Refer to Section 28d/Part c in the tax code …
• Failure to submit on time will result in …
• The deadline for compliance has been extended [Note: This is the fourth extension.]
• New eligibility standards exclude …
• When employer lives outside designated area, you must use forms …
• Improper code number submitted. Revise and re-submit no later than …
• If you answered "Yes" to question 174, fill out additional pages …
• If you have the following conditions, you may not …
• Federal guidelines require your health care provider to …
• This website is currently being revised. Please come back later.
• *Wenn sie komst sofort auf der* … [German, which you don't speak]
• Rule 1198c outside frequent registered alternate only [Gibberish, this time in English]
• Insert tab B into flange F after rotating cam L is fully seated. [Just checking to see if you are still reading, or have your eyes totally glazed over?]

Out of this miasma comes your "savior." This is the hero who will guide you out of the fog. This newly minted bureaucrat will help you through all that convoluted language and will show you the way to safety and the security of federal compliance. However, what the cancer-ridden bureaucracy hides from you is that the person now posing as your "savior" is same person who created the choking fog in the first place—a federal bureaucrat, just with a different name.

Since it would be over-the-top for the bureaucrats to call themselves heroes or saviors, the ACA created a name for them: Navigators.

The ACA created this new bureaucrat, the navigator (sometimes called in-person assister), who will help you get through the complex fog of incomprehensible forms, contradictory rules, data overload, and constant revisions. The Law requires all health exchanges to hire and fund this new position, thousands of them.

Ask yourself, why do I need a navigator? Why is the ACA so complex and constantly changing that we all need navigators? You know the answer: Purposefully created complexity gives the bureaucracy an excuse to keep expanding. Navigators are the proof.

In fact, the ACA is so complex that not even the IRS can comply with it. The IRS sent out ACA-mandated tax forms, which it turns out, were wrong. The error was only uncovered after more than eight hundred thousand Americans followed the IRS instructions, sent in their forms, were then threatened with penalties for their erroneous filings, only to discover later that it was the IRS's fault.

Apparently, even the IRS—the Gestapo of the federal bureaucracy—is caught in the fog of bureaucratic complexity. Maybe they should hire their own navigators rather than the 1,954 new hitmen (oops, sorry, agents) planned to implement the new ACA's changes in the tax code.[12]

Over six *billion* bureaucrat man-hours have already been devoted to writing new tax rules, regulations, and oversight compliance requirements. Overall, the IRS has requested more than $430 billion in new spending to implement the ACA. Remember, those are 430 billion "healthcare" dollars that produce no health care. I cannot think of a better demonstration of artificial, unnecessary, and thus wasteful intentional complexity.

If healthcare were designed to be user-friendly, we wouldn't need Navigators in the first place. If things were as simple as they should be (and could be), we would spend more "healthcare" dollars on health care (taking care of you) and less on healthcare bureaucrats.

Root Cause Revisited

Here's something I ran across on the Internet that dramatizes how most of us feel about federal bureaucrats.

> Late one night in Washington, D.C., a mugger wearing a ski mask jumps into the path of a man in an Armani suit-and-tie, and sticks a gun in his ribs.
>
> "Give me your money," the thief demands.
>
> The man puffs himself up and indignantly replied, "You can't rob ME—I work for the government. In fact, I am an IRS agent for the ACA!!"
>
> Slowly cocking the pistol, the robber steps even closer, puts the gun right in the man's face and snarls "Well, in that case you greedy S.O.B. bureaucrat, give me back *my* money that *you* stole!"

A bureaucracy is composed of bureaucrats. Professional politicians give orders to the bureaucrats. The bureaucrats interpret their orders and then carry them out.

When cancer takes over, the orders coming down from the politicians to their henchmen bureaucrats are quite simple. (1) Cancel all previous instructions. (2) Grab all the resources—money and time. (3) Grow as big as you can and wherever possible. (4) Ignore the consequences. Period.

Please note that cancer is apolitical, or should I write bipartisan? The Democrats openly say they want more government control, i.e., they want a bigger cancer with greater reach, claiming that that is how they will deliver on their entitlement assurances. We will see in chapter 9 how well they did on their Obamacare promises.

The Republicans say they want to scale back government, restore the free market, and return control to the individual, but they don't do it. They too enlarge the bureaucracy.

The cancer has taken over all of Washington, from the White House and Congress to a dizzying array of federal agencies. Cancer has reprogrammed them all to cease their proper function and simply GROW.

A recent IRS ruling makes this point dramatically.[13] You and I both thought a purpose of the Affordable Care Act was to increase the number of Americans with insurance. So how can we understand a ruling that penalizes small businesses $36,500 per year per employee if the employer pays for part or all of the employee's insurance premiums for insurance that is not ACA compliant? This makes no sense until you acknowledge the true purpose of the IRS ruling; recognize the real goal of the ACA law; and accept the true function of the federal bureaucracy: They serve the cancer, not us.

If you want to protect yourself and your family, you need to know your enemy. Cancer has taken over and reprogrammed the federal healthcare bureaucracy so that it now supports the cancer's insatiable, mindless drive to grow, and ignores the medical needs of Americans.

If there were no cancer, you could get the medical care you need when and where you need it and at a price you could afford.

Now you know the truth about the root cause. There are other facts that you may think are true, that are actually false. In the next chapter, we will examine some of this *accepted wisdom* and learn painfully that it is neither wise nor should it be accepted.

SEVEN

Myths Of BARRC

In the last chapter, I mentioned that I had coined a term for the elements that make up a bureaucracy and describe what it does: BARRC. It stands for: Bureaucracy, Administration, Rules, Regulations, and Compliance.

By now, I hope you get the idea that bureaucracy is where the malignancy resides.

This cancer is destroying the American healthcare system. BARRC is the tool by which the cancer controls us and expands itself. BARRC is so overwhelming that it makes you feel powerless, like you can't fight back.

BARRCs bite is eventually fatal, as you will see in the next chapter.

As a doctor, I have felt the bite of BARRC on a host of occasions. One such incident finally tipped me over the edge.

In the healthcare field, there is a bureaucracy known as the JCAHO Joint Commission on Accreditation of Healthcare Organizations. It is a federal agency authorized to accredit or de-license healthcare organizations: hospitals, outpatient treatment facilities, nursing homes, etc. Several years ago, they shortened the name to the Joint Commission, possibly to make it seem less threatening to healthcare organizations. (It didn't work.)

The Joint Commission visits hospitals, etc. every two to three years to judge their compliance with federal rules. Are they following the latest, revised, updated, and adjusted requirements? When they came to my institution several years ago, we were found "out of compliance." Two of the infractions were attributed to me.

What did I do wrong? Was the infection rate in my patients inordinately high? Did I operate on children while intoxicated? Did I leave a sponge in a patient? Did someone die needlessly? None of the above, thank you very much. What I did was *far* worse, at least in the eyes of the bureaucracy.

My two violations were:

1. The Joint Commission bureaucrat found a doorstop in my lab where I kept the teaching collection of heart specimens.

2. The bureaucrat, climbing up to the top of my bookshelves, discovered that the books on the top shelf in my office were too close to the ceiling tiles.

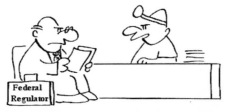

Out of compliance for "Book Too Tall"?!?

That was why the federal reviewers cited my hospital, which then was required to undergo a re-review in six months to assure that we were now "in" compliance (or else!) I made darn sure there were no doorstops anywhere and that the books on the top shelf were all within regulation.

This is God's honest truth. I cannot make up stuff like this.

I pondered over why these "regs" were in place for a hospital. Perhaps having books too close to the ceiling tiles was a fire hazard. Maybe that doorstop put my heart specimens in some sort of danger. This all might seem funny in its triviality, but the BARRC from the Joint Commission review is deadly serious business.

If a hospital or institution does not comply with all the regulations, it is in danger of losing licensure. That meant that if I didn't change the height of my books, my entire hospital could have been shut down. This is a very big *stick* and the Joint Commission knows it. They revel in the power. Their judgments— "In Compliance" or "Out of Compliance"—are questions of institutional survival. The BARRC imposed by the Joint Commission determines who gets to stay in business, who has a job, and who gets to joins the ranks of the unemployed?

Greed in the corporate healthcare world is obvious, ugly, and costs us billions of dollars. But that greed pales in comparison to the seemingly limitless appetite of BARRC. Bureaucracy wields enormous power, and the bureaucrats who create BARRC are constantly seeking more. It is profoundly disheartening to see what has happened to the great American Experiment and how our grand ideals have been degraded. Our Founding Fathers would be amazed and disgusted to see what we have done with what they gave us.

It is time to confront the issue head-on so that we can begin to do something about it.

Some still see the government with its bureaucracy as protector and savior. Others accept them as a necessary evil and something that just can't be fixed. Most do not recognize how much it costs them, both directly and indirectly. Worse, very few seem to recognize the grave danger to our individual health and to our freedom that a cancerous bureaucracy poses.

BARRC—More Poison Than Panacea

Fabio Casartelli was a twenty-five-year-old Italian cyclist and Olympic Gold medalist (1992) who was the first Tour de France racer to die from a crash (1995.)[1] No one knows why he lost control during the steep descent of the Col de Portet d'Aspet. The impact of his helmetless head against a tree cut short what was a promising career.

What impacts us when Congress passes legislation, any legislation? It is not the Act itself; that is the intention, the concept or idea. What hits us in the head (like Casartelli's tree) is the BARRC. Regardless of what the politicians say, even how the Act reads, it is BARRC that takes money out of your wallet and bites you on the … hand.

Medicaid Law says we should provide care for those unable to care for themselves. That is a nice theory, and makes everyone feel good. The practical reality is the bureaucracy establishes the eligibility requirements that defines those who are "unable to care for themselves," and bureaucrats decide who amongst those numbers actually get care, when, and how much.

BARRC is where the rubber meets the road. Sometimes, those federal rules and regulations have acted as a panacea, actually helping us. However, more commonly than not, BARRC is poison. It hurts the very people it says it will help.

As we saw in the last chapter, federal bureaucrats have brilliantly positioned themselves as our saviors, rescuing us from the very BARRC they created. There are many falsehoods that the cancer in bureaucracy has repeated and repeated until we come to believe them like, "Ignorance is strength, Freedom is slavery" (George Orwell's *1984*), with the most ridiculous being, *I'm from the government and I'm here to help.*

To protect ourselves, we must know the true truths (that should be a redundancy but sadly, it is not), rather than the false truths the cancer wants us to believe. Here are some of the myths that bureaucrats and politicians assure us are accepted wisdom. Read on and decide for yourself if what they say about BARRC is true.

Myth #1: BARRC Doesn't Cost Me Anything

After "Trust me!" the next favorite come-on line of every politician is, "This regulation or that rule won't cost you a penny!" Because we all love something that has a big ole' *FREE* sticker attached to it, we become easily blinded by the truth: every regulatory bureaucracy, whether Federal or State, generates direct costs as well as indirect costs. We pay both.

The direct cost is one that can be easily measured: paying the salaries and generous benefits of millions of bureaucrats, including their travel and other expenses from new buildings to supplies and computers. The direct cost is in the hundreds of billions of dollars per agency per year, but that figure is hidden from public scrutiny. Have you ever seen the Congressional Budget Office show the details of how much it costs to run a single bureau of the government? I certainly haven't, and I've looked ... hard.

The indirect costs are the downstream effects of rules and regulations. I do not know this cost. No one does. Indirect costs are not measured, even though they probably represent a greater expense than the direct costs.

Let me share with you one of my favorite "pet peeve" examples. I've already talked about how HIPAA requires all computers in any medical or dental office to be shielded so that passer's by cannot see what is on the screen. That is an indirect cost of BARRC. It gets worse.

Say you're Dr. J, a family practitioner. The Joint Commission inspects your office and finds that your computer screens aren't shielded properly. You have to hurry up and get in compliance, buy the necessary equipment, and be subjected to another inspection—which by the way you're billed for—because if you don't, you're office is going to be closed. The bureaucracy doesn't count all the money that you, Dr. J, have to spend to get your office in compliance. However, as I have pointed out before, Dr. J has to pass on his cost to you-the-patient. The higher office fee is an indirect cost generated by BARRC that you, the patient, must pay.

There are thousands of examples of indirect costs of BARRC. I've already pointed out that the name of the patient does not appear on the outside of hospital charts. HIPAA forbids it. How many avoidable errors are caused because of this "rule"? What is the cost in terms of adverse patient outcomes of the errors caused when a doctor orders the wrong drug for a patient or makes the wrong diagnosis because vital information was withheld or simply unavailable due to government security protocols? What about just the cost of this built-in error-promoting mandated inefficiency?

Though the huge indirect costs of regulations are not measured, they still exist. Someone has to pay them. Of course, you know that means you and me.

I cannot write that BARRC are totally worthless. I cannot determine their worth because I do not know their cost/benefit ratio. What is unforgivable is that *neither does Congress.*

Cost/benefit analysis of BARRC is unknown for three reasons. None is acceptable.

1. The Government Accounting Office does not calculate indirect costs, long-term costs, and avoided costs, so no one knows the total cost.

2. Any benefit you might receive from BARRC is purely theoretical: there is no proof that such benefits exist, none whatsoever. People in Congress simply say they exist. Typically they promise wonderful benefits, like "Under ACA, everybody will get more (health care) and pay less," per Nancy Pelosi on *Meet the Press*.[2] No one makes any attempt to prove these grandiose promises. They don't quantify the benefits to patients, to society, or to the nation, and they never, ever give us the evidence for how much they spend or where our money goes.

   We do get one thing. We get, repeatedly, "Trust me, it won't cost you anything," lawmakers said when the debates started raging over passage of the ACA bill back in 2009-2010. "Trust me that it will be good for you," they continue to chant. It baffles me how we, as a country, can keep putting our trust in lawmakers who lie, cheat, and steal, who exempt themselves from their own rules, and who never make good on their promises? Why? Why do we keep doing it?

3. Humans always think of themselves first. This is true for you and me, for care providers, and certainly for bureaucrats. But if bureaucrats did careful, accurate cost/benefit analyses of the rules and regulations they create, most of their jobs would disappear. If you and I could see how much government BARRC really costs, there would be riots in the streets.

You Get What You Reward

Finding hospitals "out of compliance," means job security for regulatory bureaucrats. This is a classic perverse incentive. It's like your car mechanic being paid more as he finds more things to fix on your car, or your doctor being paid more as you get sicker. Such perverse incentives serve only to provide job security for the auto mechanic, the doctor, and the bureaucrat.

In 1975, Steven Kerr wrote a paper that everyone should read. I do mean everyone, because it applies to all aspects of life. Its title is "On the folly of rewarding A While hoping for B."[3] Kerr talks about the obvious: when you reward outcomes differently, the person who is seeking the outcome will make sure the more attractive alternative is chosen. He uses examples from politics, war, universities, and a slew of other professional areas to prove his point.

For his medical example, Kerr relates that in 1995, in Broward County, Florida, psychiatrists were paid $325 if they found someone insane (incompetent) and $125 if they decided the person was competent and sane. Guess how many individuals were insane versus sane?

A whopping 570 out of 598 (95 percent) were declared insane! Do you think the way they were paid had anything to do with what the psychiatrists decided? That was a classic case of a perverse incentive.

In 2014, newspaper headlines in my home state of New Mexico regaled us with the fraud and abuse charges leveled against fifteen different private, non-profit organizations that provide behavioral health service for some of our neediest individuals: troubled youth, developmentally delayed, and people with major psychiatric problems.

Ignore for a moment whether the charges are true or false. Let's expose two ways that perverse incentives play right into the hands of the bureaucratic cancer.

First, New Mexico immediately stopped funding the agencies without public hearings or a trial. In fact, the allegations have been kept secret so the accused agencies are not allowed to see the evidence against them. The State has punished them as though they were proven guilty, even though they had not been afforded any opportunity to defend themselves. What happened to "due process" (Fifth Amendment to the U.S. Constitution)?

Why is the bureaucracy behaving this way? "To protect the best interests of our most vulnerable," it was *forced* to take control of these agencies. Thus, BARRC expands and extends its reach, and thrusts bureaucrats directly into making medical decisions for mental-health patients. That's really scary.

Second, you need to know how the evidence was acquired to *convict* these agencies (without a trial). An outside accounting firm was contracted by the State to review the agencies' administrative practices and money flow. Here's the telling part. The accounting firm was paid according to how many charges of fraud they reported and how much money they could claim the accused agencies had embezzled or misused. So the more fraud and abuse they reported (not proved, just claimed), the more money they made.

No wonder the fifteen agencies were accused of misusing $34 million. The reviewer got a piece of the action. Great way to get at the truth, isn't it?

What incentive is there for a healthcare regulatory compliance officer to find any hospital in compliance … *ever*? The bureaucrat only receives a reward (more power and better job security) if he finds a hospital *out* of compliance. When he approves the hospital, he proves that he and his agency are no longer needed.

If you want to avoid such perverse incentives, remember this: You get what you *reward,* not what you want, and certainly not what you deserve.[4] So instead of sitting back and thinking that the lawmakers in Washington are taking good care of us, look at current legislation in Congress. See for yourself if these laws create more and more bureaucracy, and if that bureaucracy helps us or helps only itself. And, most important, we should demand that legislators give us evidence-based cost/benefit analyses before they pass new laws.

Libertarian P.J. O'Rourke quipped, "Giving money and power to government [especially over two trillion dollars a year for healthcare] is like giving whiskey and car keys to teenage boys."[5]

Myth #2: BARRC Reduces Costs

One of the biggest gripes about healthcare is the high cost of health insurance premiums. Their un-affordability was the initial justification for ACA. Congress thought that excessive premiums were the reason that forty-five million Americans were uninsured. They called this a national disgrace. So, our "ultimate ally" Congress, *had* to step in to make healthcare "affordable" for all. Enter Obamacare.

The president promised he would make health care so affordable, that it would be free! Somehow—with lots of media help to be sure—people got the idea that everyone could have insurance and get care without anyone paying anything extra.

The BARRC in Obama's ACA was touted to reduce the cost of insurance by controlling those greedy insurance companies who profit at our expense. His "reform" was said to be good for everyone ... well, apparently not everyone. There were some notable exceptions—groups that were promised exemptions from a law that was supposed to help everyone. It was our first clue that something was not right.

First, union supporters of the president were granted exemptions. Then, certain religious groups were added to the list.[6] Of course, ACA did not apply to illegal residents, who still received "free" care under EMTALA.[7] The list of exemptions quickly became longer and longer until there were over fourteen hundred groups and organizations for whom the so-called "benefits" of ACA *reform* did not apply.

Then, Congressmen and women began to say they too had to be exempt. Their explanation was fascinating. The reason given for Congress opting out of their own plan was that it Obamacare was too costly for congressional staffers.[8] Wait a minute! Wasn't the whole point to make insurance more affordable for the average American, not more prohibitively expensive?

Next, the union for the IRS agents (NTEU, National Treasury Employees Unions) started griping that Obamacare wasn't good for them because of all the extra costs they would have to pay. Apparently, they just discovered what most Americans suspected: Obama's "affordable care" wasn't affordable and certainly wasn't fair to the average hard working, tax-paying American.[9]

It's Just A Tax, Ma'am

Things really started getting squirrely when the bureaucracy began implementing Obamacare. We learned that care wasn't "free" at all, and that we were penalized by something called the Individual Mandate if we chose not to buy insurance. It wasn't a tax, promised the President, until SCOTUS chimed in on the matter.

In 2012, the Supreme Court of the United States (SCOTUS) struck down the individual mandate in ACA: it was unconstitutional.[10] But the Chief Justice then explained that the mandate could be kept—if it changed its name to a tax. So the tax President Obama swore wasn't a tax became a tax.

Now that Obamacare is a reality, does it make health insurance affordable or not?

In New York State, a family of four earning $35,000 will have to spend $5,555 a year—16 percent of their total gross (pre-tax) income—to pay for ObamaCare health insurance.[11] No one would ever call that "affordable." Before ACA, average annual cost for the same family was $1728/year.

Say the New York family is better off and earns $85,000 per year. What is their cost? They will pay $16,408 (19 percent) per year in total health care expenditures as a result of ObamaCare.

What about effects of ACA on costs to employers?

The penalty for not offering insurance to employees is a tiny fraction of what an employer's increased cost of procuring employee insurance under ACA. What do you think employers will do? Well, they have already begun doing it: cutting work hours so people become part-time (and therefore not eligible for health benefits).[12] Other employers aren't hiring at all or even terminating. As an adverse and unintended (we presume) consequence of ACA, men and women who want to work but cannot find a job are forced to eek out an existence on day labor and live in homeless shelters.[13] Putting extremes aside, more and more employers are simply cancelling health insurance for their employees. If they try to pay the increased ACA costs, they cannot make payroll.

A Robert Wood Johnson Foundation report showed the effects of ACA in California.[14] Compared to 2009 (before ACA) over a million *fewer* Californians are now getting their health insurance at work. Why? Because they can't! It's not offered, they no longer qualify, or they simply cannot afford it.

The PCIP (Pre-Existing Condition Insurance Plan (see chapter 2) is another demonstration of the cruel myth that "ACA will make insurance affordable for all." Let me relate what was said at a recent Board meeting of the New Mexico Health Insurance Exchange.

One member of the Board had unfortunate news to report in his position as Chairman of our state's High Risk Insurance Pool. This covers roughly ten thousand New Mexicans, all American citizens, who have serious chronic illnesses (read: expensive pre-existing conditions) and cannot get insurance through the standard market. No one will insure them because insurers know their medical costs are enormous. In 2013, those 10,000 people cost our state roughly two hundred million dollars for their health care.

As part of President Obama's promise to cover the uninsured and uninsurable, ACA created PCIP, which was a pool of five billion dollars that they said would cover all the medical needs for an estimated 365,000 uninsurable Americans. Within two years all that money had been used up, not providing care but creating bureaucracy. Approximately, 125,000 individuals had signed up when Washington stopped enrollment, leaving 240,000 people out in the cold.[15]

Our Board member regretfully reported all this to us, including the fact that his 10,000 citizens could not sign up for PCIP and thus were left stranded with no health insurance. They would have to come into the general insurance pool, which would certainly raise the insurance rates the Exchange could offer, possibly returning to the un-affordable range. "ACA affordable insurance" is more than just a false promise—it's turning into a cruel, taunting mirage.

Washington is spending money by the trillions. If it is not making insurance affordable, what is it doing?

The money is being spent to expand the bureaucracy. In New Mexico, the Health Exchange Board first year's spending was $54,282,927. Not one of those dollars went to a patient. All of it went to comply with federal implementation requirements.

Put yourself in the shoes of a resident of New York, Massachusetts, or California. (Maybe you are already in them.) You can no longer get insurance at work if you are lucky enough to have a full-time job.

Before Obamacare, you couldn't afford insurance. Now it is even more expensive.

Meanwhile, you will have to pay the ACA penalty ("tax" according to the U.S. Supreme Court) for not having insurance. This will cost you $695 per person by 2016 (and you're still not insured.) For the families of four in New York, that translates to $2780 per year if you do not purchase Obama's insurance compared to $5,555 to $16, 408 if you do.

Is this what we were promised? Apparently not. Again I refer you to the unions for proof. Kinsey Robinson, President of the United Union of Roofers, WaterProofers and Allied Workers International, said, "I refuse to remain silent, or idly watch as the ACA destroys those protections."[16] He is referring to the "protection" of union workers from all the additional costs, penalties, and taxes that are part of the ACA. The President promised the unions (along with many others) special protected status in order to get their support for both ACA and his re-election.

Myth #3: BARRC Will Control Healthcare's Over-Spending

Big Lies are falsehoods that people say the loudest and most often. A Big Lie is spoken with such authority and certitude that if you question it, you look ignorant. Unless you have the courage of the young boy in the story of the Emperor's New Clothes, you don't say, "Wait a minute, the Emperor is naked," when the Big Lie is uttered.[17]

One very Big Lie is this: You and I need all those bureaucratic controls and tight regulations—BARRC—to keep a check on the greedy corporate bast**ds who are stealing our health care (service) dollars.

In the early 1980s, there was national uproar over unnecessary duplication of expensive medical technologies as a cause of our national over-spending on healthcare. Compared to the bureaucratic greed that was in full swing even back then, this waste was quite minor, but it made national headlines. "MRI scanners on every block." "Cardiac cath labs in tiny hospitals." "CAT scans for headaches."

Because those multi-million dollar machines generated huge fees, too many of them were built, raising the cost of healthcare. The solution implemented by Congress was the C.O.N. process (Certificate

Of Need, not the other kind of "con" even though I've always found the abbreviation ironic.) Hospitals had to file statements proving their "need" to obtain a license for all the big-ticket items they want.

You probably don't need to guess what happened. It was a page out of New York City with its Tammany Hall and something called a "little tin box." This was a song from the 1959 hit musical *Fiorello!* about Mayor Fiorella H. LaGuardia. The tin box referred to the hiding place where government officials would put their proceeds from graft, corruption, and underhanded dealings. For your enjoyment, I have copied one stanza and the chorus.

> [Stanza] "Mr. Y, we've been told you don't feel well,
> And we know you've lost your voice,
> But we wonder how you managed on the salary you make
> To acquire a new Rolls-Royce."
> "You're implyin' I'm a crook and I say no, sir!
> There is nothin' in my past I care to hide.
> I been takin' empty bottles to the grocer
> And each nickel that I got was put aside."
> (That he got was put aside.)
> [Chorus] "Into a little tin box,
> A little tin box
> That a little tin key unlocks.
> There is nothing unorthodox
> About a little tin box.
> In a little tin box,
> A little tin box
> There's a cushion for life's rude shocks.
> There is faith, hope and charity,
> Hard-won prosperity,
> In a little tin box."

If you are from the Southwest or from California, the phrase you know is "pay to play," meaning money under the table that gets you regulatory approval. If you want your expensive machines, you pay the bureaucrats under the table and amazingly, your C.O.N. is approved.

That is how the New Mexico State Employee Pension Fund lost tens of millions of dollars: crony capitalism, under-the-table deals, with our money ending up in "little tins boxes" held by New York friends of the former Governor of New Mexico.[18]

Did C.O.N. legislation, another manifestation of BARRC, reduce duplication of medical services? No, it did not. Did it cut spending on healthcare? Quite the opposite. C.O.N. filings greatly increased spending on healthcare bureaucracy, especially by augmenting the salaries of bureaucrats, lawyers, PR firms, actuaries, and lobbyists. Someone had to pay them. Of course, that "someone" is the same someone who pays all the bills: You and me, We The Patients.

Myth #4: BARRC Are Always Good For Us

Of all the insidious myths about BARRC, this one is the cherry on top. This *accepted wisdom* says that BARRC are always beneficial. This myth implies that BARRC never produce unexpected, unintended, or adverse consequences. I don't know who really believes that, but our lawmakers and their partners-in-crime, the bureaucrats, simply make that assertion and assume that no one will question it—that is, not until we start looking, for ourselves, at the evidence.

To judge any outcome, you should ask yourself four questions. (1) Who had what *expectations*? (2) Who had which *intentions*? (3) Since "adverse" means harm, who was *harmed*, and how? (4) Don't forget Joseph Stalin's favorite question of all, "Who benefits?"[19]

ACA, as always, provides an excellent demonstration case. We shall answer the four questions from two perspectives: the union supporters of ACA (whom I will call "us" in this instance), and the bureaucratic cancer.

As I noted above, the unions expected that ACA would not raise their members' insurance premiums, and for certain, they expected they could keep their employer-supported health insurance. Unions had a right to expect this because that is what the President promised them. The bureaucracy, on the other hand, expected ACA to raise large sums of money so it could grow.

Guess what? Union members, like everyone else, are facing increased insurance premium costs. To whom are the effects of ACA "adverse" in this instance? Who was harmed and how? The unions quite rightly feel that they were harmed by the President's "untruth." Millions of union members, like other employees in America, discover that paying the ACA penalty is much cheaper than their health insurance premiums.

The effects of ACA—people losing everything from their healthcare benefits to their jobs—are not unexpected, are not unintended, and certainly are not adverse from the perspective of the cancer of bureaucratic greed. The cancer benefits, hugely!

For the cancer, ACA is a huge success! Government bureaucracy will be able to gather untold billions, probably trillions, in penalties and taxes. They are basically getting a windfall of more than one trillion dollars (>$1,000,000,000,000) to expand the bureaucracy—which was the cancer's desired outcome all along.

Expectation, intention, and help-or-harm are in the eye of the beholder. I hope you remember that next time you experience one of the "unexpected," "unintended," or worst of all, "adverse" effects when BARRC bites you.

Myth #5: We Need BARRC To Protect Us

The new grade school principal was checking over his school. It was his first day on the job.

While walking around, he was startled to see the stockroom door wide open and unguarded. Teachers were bustling in and out carrying off books and supplies in preparation for the arrival of students the next day. The school where he had been assistant principal the previous year had a checkout system that combined the checkout system of Fort Knox with the security protocols of nuclear silos.

Cautiously, he walked up to the school's long time custodian and asked, "Do you think it's wise to keep the stock room unlocked and to let the teachers take whatever they want without authorization and requisitions?"

The Custodian looked at him, thought for a moment, and gravely asked, "We trust them with the children, don't we?"

Do you believe that you need "protection" from your doctor? Such protection is part of the justification for BARRC, particularly the "RC" part: Regulations, Compliance, and their oversight.

Federal rules *require* every triage nurse to ask every patient who enters a doctor's office three questions. 1) "What is your pain level today?" 2) "Is anyone smoking in your house?" And 3) "Have you given any thought to suicide?" What does "thoughts of suicide" have to do with your doctor treating your physical illness? Absolutely nothing. Worse, it takes two to three minutes for the nurse to ask these questions, including documentation of the answers. If you're barely conscious from the pain or are experiencing heart-attack-like symptoms, aren't you more worried about getting the problem handled? But the questions are there to "protect you." The government is afraid that your doctor would forget to ask these "vitally important" queries, so these questions are mandated by federal law.

I had a pulmonary embolus (blood clot in the lungs) shortly after racing in the 2004 Veteran's National Track Cycling Championships.[20] As a result, I needed to have special x-rays done of my lungs. Each time, I have to fill out forms (the same form each time) that included questions about when my last menstrual period occurred, had I had a pregnancy test, and was I aware of the risks of radiation (as well as cigarette smoking!) on my growing baby? By federal law, everyone must answer these questions, every time, even if you are a male or are pre-pubescent. Talk about a waste of time and money, but BARRC demands it, so we do it.

Magazines and newspapers love to tell you how your doctor is not paying attention to you and may be harming you. Given all you learned, from whom do you need more protection: your doctor or government BARRC?

Myth #6: BARRC Assures Medical Quality

You may believe that providers who follow all the rules, regulations, and standard procedures deliver high quality, error-free care. It is natural to presume that with all those forms and guidelines, BARRC assures that We The Patients will "live long and prosper."

There is no, repeat, *no* data to prove that compliance with regulations produces better patient outcomes.

In the last fifteen years, care providers have begun to develop clinical algorithms for many common ailments. These are clinical plans for patients that have been proven scientifically to produce better outcomes. Does the government adopt them as part of their rules and regulations for doctors? No, that would make too much sense. Take the example of several intensive care units in Michigan.

They collaborated on a checklist, like a pilot's pre-flight checklist, to reduce infections in hospitalized patients. In eighteen months, their checklist saved over fifteen hundred lives and saved $200 million. The Federal government prohibited them from using the checklist because their research was not done according to standard rules and regulations.[21]

Research has proven that most heart attack patients do better afterward if they take a medicine called a beta-blocker. This drug controls heart rhythm and lowers blood pressure. At discharge from hospital, the now-accepted clinical algorithm recommends that patients receive a beta-blocker to take at home, but many don't continue the drug.

Then there is Mr. Stan Hampton, a fifty-six-year old Army veteran who had a heart attack and was admitted to his nearby VA hospital. They did a cardiac catheterization and successfully opened the blocked coronary artery without surgery. Nonetheless, Hampton had some heart damage and was clearly in the group that would benefit from a beta-blocker. At discharge, he was given a two-week supply and told to refill his medication faithfully. At follow-up six weeks later, he informed his doctors that he had stopped taking his medication when the initial bottle ran out.

The above scenario is so common that the Veterans Administration for Hospitals did a study to discover why patients were being non-compliant and not taking their medications. The reasons were numerous: too many forms to fill out, too expensive, refills denied (because, for instance, a change of address), a generic but not identical drug was substituted, the drug interacted badly with other drugs that patients were taking and therefore some pharmacists urged patients not to take the beta-blocker, patients could not get transportation to the pharmacy, even, "They just taste awful."

All those regulations and rules that supposedly protect us do the exact opposite. The regulatory system is not designed to produce what *we* want: good health. Rather, it protects their hide.

Myth #6A: BARRC Guarantees Good Medical Outcomes

The next myth is really an offshoot of #6. Because it deserves consideration on its own, I labeled it #6A. This myth suggests that complying with all the rules and regulations directly leads to error-free medical care and perfect patient outcomes. My best response is an expletive used by Col. Potter in the T.V. show, *M*A*S*H*: "Horsefeathers!"

Do you want to watch your health care provider's blood pressure go through the roof? First tell her that if she follows all the rules and regulations, she will be practicing good medicine. Then say, "If you are compliant with all the BARRC, you will fix my health problem, guaranteed." The doctor or nurse may throw up on your shoes or have a stroke. Here's what happened one early Sunday morning, 2:30 a.m.:

An ED (Emergency Dept.) physician called me about an eleven-year-old girl named CM. She was having a rapid heart rate (188 beats/minute) that started as she was going to bed two hours after soccer practice the previous evening. The ambulance team who brought her in had documented her abnormal heart rhythm on an electrocardiogram (ECG) strip.

During transport, an ambulance nurse asked her to bear down while the electrocardiogram was still running. The child's rapid rhythm converted to normal at ninety beats/minute. Thus, there was documentation of what was wrong and how it became "right." CM was admitted to hospital for observation and tests.

When I evaluated her in her hospital bed, the ECG strips were nowhere to be found. The Emergency Services tech refused to give the hospital their records saying HIPAA regulations prohibited it. An ED physician had copied some of the strips "for her own interest" but refused to share them with me because she feared that she would be Out Of Compliance with Federal confidentiality protocols and could lose her license.

How can I assure that my patient is going to have error-free healthcare when BARRC doesn't allow me access to all the information I need to treat her? How can I give her quality care when BARRC is focused solely on compliance and doesn't care what happens to my patient?

Everyone proclaims that patient care comes first but if you've ever had to deal with BARRC firsthand, you know the truth. Whatever the original intent, the effect of Federal statutes is to prioritize regulatory compliance above patient outcomes and to compel health care providers to withhold information from other providers in the name of confidentiality.

How many medical errors have been caused by federal regulations that prevent care providers from talking to each other? I do not know, but the number is large, and every single one was avoidable.

Providers are forbidden from emailing consults to other providers because, "The Internet is not secure, but the mail system is." If you believe that, I would love to sell you a bridge (to nowhere) and a swamp in Florida.

For most healthcare workers, federal regulations are effectively written on stone tablets and brought down from Mount Sinai. The worst sin is being out of compliance.

I thought about hanging the sign below on my office wall but never did. I was afraid that the next government review might declare my hospital Out Of Compliance due to my cheeky insubordination.

Compliance Beats
Medical Science
Every Time

In chapter 5, I pointed out that all practicing physicians must spend time reading government-approved online study modules on a host of subjects. Only a tiny handful of these modules have anything to do with the day-to-day practice of medicine. Yet, we have to study everything the federal bureaucracy tells us to and then pass tests on that information. If we do not, we will be Out Of Compliance, and risk the attendant fines or even losing a license to practice.

If you think I'm being overly dramatic, observe the following list of my Federally mandated "Learning Plan" for just one three-month period. I had to study each topic, take online tests, fill out forms to prove that I passed the tests, and finally, I had to get the signed forms approved by the Compliance Oversight Officer.

Not only are most of the topics unrelated to my work, but studying them took me away from actually doing what I needed to do to keep my patients alive and well. Here's the list:

- Abuse and Domestic Violence Awareness
- Basic Annual Safety Training, Revised
- Cost Measures and Public Reporting
- Ethics: A Framework for Ethical Decision Making
- HIPAA and Breach Notification—New Rules
- HIPAA and Accounting of Disclosures
- Security Guidelines, Revised
- HSC Culture of Compliance, Revised
- Anticoagulation Safety, Optimization and Compounding Sterile Preparations

- New anti-tuberculosis antibiotics—interactions and side-effects
- Smoking cessation programs
- Patient Safety
- Dealing with depression
- Preventing Sexual Harassment.

The list above was just for the first quarter of the year. There were more required study modules in the second, third, and fourth quarters.

Multiply the total time wastage by six million—the number of nurses, doctors, and allied health personnel in the U.S. The likely cost, in terms of money, is in the hundreds of billions. The cost is incalculable in terms of frustration as well as the time taken away from you and your care. Now, assess the data that shows how much benefit you get for all that time and money. That is a trick question: there is no such data.

You now understand what I mean when I say there is no evidence that proves the benefits of BARRC. If you ask the people who wrote the rules and regulations to give you their proof of effect, they will respond with, "Trust me!" (Try it sometime and let me know if I'm wrong.)

Brenner Beats BARRC

Dr. Joel Brenner, a general physician in Camden, N.J., never intended to change national healthcare policy. He certainly never thought about myth 6A. He simply wanted to practice the best medicine he could and make his patients well.

Dr. Brenner not only proved that BARRC gets in the way of good patient care. He also showed that BARRC wastes money—money that should be used for care but disappears because the bureaucracy takes it first.[22] Here's what happened:

Dr. Brenner wanted to be the best doctor he could. To him, that meant doing everything in his power to turn sick patients into healthy people. He and his Coalition for Health chose the sickest thirty-six patients they could find in Camden, New Jersey and worked to make them as healthy as possible, doing whatever it took.

To the Coalition, "whatever it took," meant practicing the best medicine possible, not following the rules. Sometimes, the providers had to ignore, adjust, re-interpret, or even subvert BARRC to do the best thing possible for the patients.

The thirty-six patients had various combinations of the most serious chronic illnesses: diabetes, chronic lung disease, heart failure, kidney failure, and multiple infections including HIV. When the Coalition took over their care, those thirty-six patients averaged sixty-seven hospital days or ER visits per month. They were generating hospital bills over $1.2 million per month!

The providers in the Coalition did anything and everything to improve patient health. BARRC required heart-failure medications to be prescribed when a patient left the hospital. One of Brenner's team went with the patient to the pharmacy to make sure they got the right medication, and knew how and when to take it. Though BARRC often allowed substitution of an alternative drug, the Coalition made sure the patients got exactly what the doctor ordered.

Multiple times per day, a colleague of Brenner would have to argue with an insurance rep or insurance Medical Director to get a patient precisely what the patient needed, when the patient needed it.

BARRC dictated that patients with breathing problems while asleep receive sleep apnea machines. Coalition nurses made home visits late at night when the patients were preparing for bed to assure that the patients applied the equipment properly and that the machines were working as necessary.

BARRC gave diabetic patients instruction papers on how and when to check their blood sugar and how to adjust insulin based on the readings. Someone from the Coalition made house calls several times per day to confirm that everything was being done correctly.

BARRC says that doctors must communicate clearly with their patients. Coalition members made sure that the patients actually understood what their doctors were saying.

The Camden Coalition focused on the end product—patient health—instead of complying with BARRC. The results were spectacular.

The patients were remarkably healthier. This translated into dramatic cost reductions. There was a 40 percent drop in hospital/ER visits. Recall that these thirty-six patients alone were previously costing $1.2 million per month. By spending approximately $50,000 per month, the Coalition reduced that $1.2 million to just over $500,000.

That calculation is worth repeating. By avoiding BARRC and while spending an additional $50,000 per month, the healthcare system (that's you and me) saved (did not have to spend) $700,000 per month. For all you investors out there, that is a 1,400 percent return on your money.

And oh by the way, the patients were also feeling much better, thank you very much.

To put it bluntly, complying with BARRC makes us sicker and costs us barrels of money. Brenner proved that. Unfortunately, the cancer in bureaucracy doesn't want to listen to these kinds of success stories. Of course, Dr. Brenner's health-promoting as well as cost-saving approach is not standard or even well known—that would put the bureaucracy at risk. Healthy happy patients and empty hospitals would make most of the bureaucracy and its BARRC unnecessary. Bureaucrats would have to join the rest of us in the unemployment lines—what a concept!

Myth #7: BARRC's Complexity Is Not Our Problem

This myth claims that the complexity that comes with BARRC is inevitable and unavoidable, but is not dangerous. Management experts, experienced engineers, wise designers, and anyone who has had to deal with an overwhelming degree of bureaucratic complexity would disagree.

Leonardo da Vinci, probably the greatest innovator in human history, said, "Simplicity is the ultimate sophistication."[23] In the previous chapter, I talked about natural complexity versus intentional complexity. The point to remember here is that *intentional* complexity gets expensive, and is used by bureaucrats in order to control those they regulate. Complexity is not intended to help us or to save money.

For contrast, the military fully understands the dangers of complexity and the compelling need for simplicity. Anything that is complex costs more, is likely to break down, and may be slow to act or react. In battlefield situations, complexity means soldiers die. That is why they simplify everything, including the organizational structure. You know precisely who is above you and who is below you. To execute an order, you don't need to study, research, interpret, think, or check the book of rules. You can act, instantly.

Compare the organizational charts of, say, the U.S. Marines, General Electric, Southwest Airlines, or Toyota to federal agencies like Medicare or the FDA (Federal Drug Administration). Count up the number of layers, then the number of boxes in each layer, and the people within each box.

The chart that follows represents the organizational structure of healthcare's bureaucracy now with ACA added. If you don't understand it, don't worry. The people who built it and even those who work within it, they don't understand it either.

What you do need to know is that all those boxes within boxes and circles connected to other circles are whole agencies with hundreds to tens of thousands of employees. Looks unnecessarily complex. It is … and you pay for all of it.

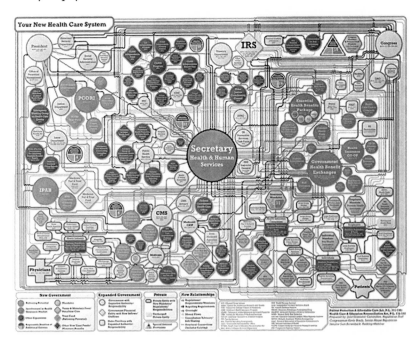

When you think about the difference between federal organizational charts and the business ones, it is truly frightening. Why does it scare me? Because we can't afford it and we are not getting the service we need. We are consistent losers. But there is one invariable winner: the cancer.

Columnist Nick Gillespie recently wrote, "When government fails, it expands. The worse it fails, the faster it expands."[24] Healthcare is experiencing an unprecedented failure, and our government is therefore experiencing an unprecedented explosion in size. One obvious indicator is that public sector (government) jobs are being advertised all over the Web. Every day, at least twice a day, I get emails with subject lines like, "Public Service Jobs in Healthcare." These are not advertisements for people who actually provide health care.

When the cancerous healthcare bureaucracy expands, it takes resources needed by its host. The host is We The Patients. Instead of a government that is spending "by and for the people," we have BARRC that is spending *by* the bureaucracy *on* the bureaucracy.

Even when confronted with the fact that eventually its host—we the taxpayers—will die from starvation, the cancer doesn't care. It keeps growing and justifies that growth by saying we need them—the bureaucrats—to help us deal with the increasing complexity. Who, might I ask, created that complexity in the first place?

This joke (modified) that I found on the Internet sums things up nicely.

Recently, a large government bureaucracy hired several cannibals to increase their diversity. "You are all part of our team now," said the Human Resources rep during the welcoming briefing. "You get all the usual benefits and you can go to the cafeteria for something to eat, but please, please don't eat any employees."

The cannibals promised they would not.

Four weeks later their boss remarked, "You're all working very hard and I'm satisfied with your work. We have noticed a marked increase in the whole company's performance. However, one of our secretaries has disappeared. Do any of you know what happened to her?"

The cannibals looked at each other and all shook their heads, "No."

After the boss had left, the leader of the cannibals said to the others, "Which one of you idiots ate the secretary?" A hand rose hesitantly.

"You fool!" the leader continued. "For four weeks we've been eating managers and no one even noticed. But now, you had to go and spoil it all by eating someone who actually does some work."

Final Myth: Single Payer Will Save Us

Upon entering a local restaurant last week, my wife and I ran into another couple we know who also work in healthcare. They joined us for dinner and the conversation inevitably turned to the ACA. My friend's wife said it was clear that Obamacare was not performing as promised but that was okay. She believed that when ACA collapsed, we would all get what she (and President Obama) wanted all along—single payer.

I asked her what she meant by single payer and why she thought it was a good idea. Her answer reflects what some people mistakenly think is the single payer option. She replied, "The government will pay our medical bills. There will be no more obscene insurance company profits and administrative costs will go way down. We can use all that money to pay to get the health care we need when we need it."

First, we need to be clear what a single payer system is. Then we will consider what it does and how it works.[25]

Single payer refers to any system in which the federal government, not the individual and not an insurance carrier, pays for health care activities. Revenue is obtained centrally, usually through taxes. The government decides how much to pay for goods and services. There are no free market forces and thus, there is no incentive to economize. In single payer, there is no commercial profit. Note that I specified *commercial* profit.

Single payer does away with insurance company denials and appeals. It eliminates the obscene profits of insurance executives and pharmaceutical conglomerates. Advocates say it streamlines the administration of healthcare.

Does it?

We already have our own, homegrown, single payer system: the Veterans Administration (VA) Hospitals. If you read a newspaper or watched TV during 2014, you know the continuing health care disaster that our veterans suffer. They are literally dying while waiting on line for "approved" medical care. The VA single-payer system has failed those for whom it is supposed to care.

The group called the Physicians For a National Health Program (PNHP) is an advocacy group that believes single payer will save us. Their website clearly states why they believe this.[26] When their promises are compared to the hard evidence from other countries who have single payer systems, you can decide for yourself whether single payer is our savior or not.

Following are a series of quotes from their website followed by facts:

"Each person, regardless of the ability to pay, would receive high-quality comprehensive medical care, and free choice of doctors and hospitals."

In Canada and Great Britain patients are assigned to medical panels and health care institutions by the government. They do not have "free choice of doctors and hospitals."

Delaying my British mum's hip replacement surgery (chapter 5) for over two years was what the British NHS called "high-quality comprehensive care." In the video "Sick and Sicker" about the Canadian system, you hear story after story of medical therapies denied, not available, or not available in time to help the patient. This is certainly not what you would call high quality or comprehensive care.

Two patients limp in to two different medical clinics, both complaining of trouble walking due to severe pain in a hip. Two different doctors suspect they need the same approach: hip replacement.

The first patient's doctor is a general physician who refers the patient to a specialist, who can see the patient in two months—eight weeks of continuous pain and virtual immobility. When the patient finally gets in, the orthopedic surgeon orders x-rays and an MRI. They are scheduled for two weeks and five weeks hence respectively, at facilities in different parts of the city. When the tests are done, the patient limps back into the surgeon's office where the doctor says, "Your primary doctor was right. You need hip replacement. I can do it in six weeks. It will cost $45,000 and insurance will pay sixty percent. Do you want me to schedule it? If so, the hospital will need a deposit of $18,000."

The second patient is examined within an hour of entering the office, X-rayed there (then), and has surgery scheduled for the following week. Cost = $2000.

What is the difference? The first patient is a U.S. veteran whose care is provided by our own, home grown single payer system. The second patient is a Labrador retriever.

The PNHP website claims:

> "95% of people would pay less for health care ... would save billions, and could be redistributive."

No one is sure whether it was Mark Twain or Benjamin Disraeli who uttered those five immortal words: "Lies, damned lies, and statistics." Whoever said it could have been referring to the quote above.

The use of a number, especially one as high as "95%," suggests reliability and accuracy. However, it diverts your attention away from the truth. Ninety-five percent of people in single payer do not simply pay "less." They pay *nothing* for their health care, directly that is. They pay money to the government and the government pays their health care bills.

Unfortunately, as I have shown over and over, the government first takes its "cut" for all its BARRC. What is left over becomes available for your care. So, while people pay nothing *directly* in single payer, they pay quite a great deal indirectly, much more than they would if government were not involved.

In Alberta, Canada, the Minister for Health reported that forty percent of the entire Provincial budget was consumed by healthcare. Remember who gets first crack at those dollars. It isn't care services for Canadians.

How does the single payer "save" all those billions?[27] Answer: by issuing new rules, regulations, and guidelines, i.e., by adding even more BARRC (and remember, BARRC costs money.)

PNHP claims that:

"Slashing to Canadian levels [of administrative spending] would save ... enough to cover the uninsured."

You really have to question the sanity of anyone who believes that expanding government control (of anything!) saves money. I defy such a person to show any instance, a single one, where an increase in BARRC resulted in reduced spending.

Government control, as in a single payer system, will dramatically raise costs. Scary as that is, there is something worse. As the government spends **your** money on **it**self, there is not enough left to provide your health care. So, single payers "save" money by denying you the care you need.

As for saving "enough to pay for the uninsured," that too is distortion. In single payer, there are no uninsured, except of course for non-citizens. While not a big problem in Canada, there are twelve to fifteen million "illegal" Americans. In Germany, there are over two million Turkish guest workers. Under single payer, these "uninsured" individuals would be denied care.

More on the myth about single payer promoted by PNHP:

"Single payer is the only plan which features effective cost control measures."

I could laugh except that I am crying (for my patients).

Under single payer, those so-called "effective cost control measures" have nothing to do with the cost of your care. These measures are effective in balancing the budget, not getting you the care you need when you need it at a reasonable cost. Let's call these cost controls what they are: medical rationing.

In Great Britain, the medical rationing agency is called N.I.C.E. (talk about ironic acronyms), which stands for National Institute for

Clinical Excellence. ACA's Independent Advisory Payment Board was modeled on NICE. Both are government agencies tasked with balancing expenditures for healthcare—both the system and the service—with the national budget. Your medical needs are irrelevant.

Here is an example. Imagine that you are a 56-year old British citizen and your kidneys are failing. Dialysis would save your life. You cannot get it as *your* NHS denies authorization. It has decreed that kidney dialysis over the age of 55 years is "Not Cost Effective." You could go on living if you paid approximately $10,000/month for your own, private dialysis. That's in Great Britain. In Canada, the single payer Law prohibits you from paying, even if you have the money.

You can decide what you consider "effective cost control measures." Speaking for all physicians, any law that prevents us from giving optimal care to our patients is unconscionable and against every medical code of ethics I know.

PNHP can be frankly disingenuous:

"Budgets for capital [expenditures] would be based on healthcare priorities."

"Healthcare priorities" refer to priorities for the government, not priorities for patients. Balancing the budget comes before patient health care needs.

When the U.S. VA scandal hit the front pages, what did Congress do? It suddenly *found* $17 billion to give to the VA. Where were they for years when veterans died needlessly waiting to see a doctor? Only the political pressure, not the highest-priority patients' needs, made them act. (And VA problems persist, despite all that "found" money.)[28]

In the next chapter, you will read about Dr. Ciaran McNamee who showed how Canada's single payer budgeting process left providers with too few operating rooms, and too little medicine to provide the care that patients need, when they need it.

Years ago, there was a blog from Australia (another single payer) titled, "If I stayed in Australia, I'd be dead now." It was written by a woman reporter who developed a rare form of breast cancer, one that responded only to a new therapy. The government of Australia deemed the treatment Not Cost Effective as well as Experimental and rejected her doctor's request to use it. It was, however, the only treatment that would save her. She left "down under," got the medicine, and lived to write the story.

Ask any Canadian, Briton, or American veteran this question: who gets the first and biggest bite of the healthcare dollar—their health care needs or the maw of bureaucracy? Watch out. They might throw something at you.

We have dispelled a number of comforting but totally false myths about BARRC. So now you ask, "But Dr. Deane, is BARRC really so bad? A lot of red tape and some unnecessary spending, but is it actually dangerous to me?"

I must answer, "Yes, it is quite dangerous." In fact, healthcare BARRC is shaping up to be lethal.

EIGHT

When Bureaucracy Becomes Lethal

"Feed the bureaucracy. Divert the money from providers to bureaucrats." This is the mantra that the cancer instills, prompting politicians to make decisions that can be lethal to all non-bureaucrats.

In people, cancer cells kill normal cells by starving them: the cancer diverts resources that the normal cells need to live and to function. So, for example, when cancer takes energy from heart muscle cells, guess what happens?

In our healthcare system, cancer has spread to all parts of the bureaucracy. It has taken control so it can grow. Cancer grows by sucking the life out of those it feeds on: That's us, We The Patients.

If we do not stop the cancer, healthcare bureaucracies will move from passively killing us to actively doing so. In effect, the bureaucracy is becoming our executioner. If you believe that is paranoid craziness, look at what is happening right now in Great Britain with its Liverpool Care Protocol, something I will discuss later in this chapter.

For now, know that there are a number of ways in which the cancerous bureaucracy is pushing us toward the grave in order to keep itself alive. The irony of this should now be clear: The bureaucracy needs our dollars for it to survive, but the cancer is choking off the very thing it needs to live. This is why it is lethal.

I must warn you: Bureaucrats couch the danger you're in by using positive remarks like,

- "It's in your own best interest."
- "Trust me!"
- "The budget will not allow that" (the care you need to stay alive.)
- "This will ease your suffering."
- "We have to consider the greater good."

These are all code for "we want more of your money even though we know it takes away from your care." Don't expect the bureaucracy to want to spend money on us for our health care. Regardless of whether it is the corporate bureaucracy or the government bureaucracy who steals the most, the consequences of starving the "care" part of healthcare cannot be ignored.

Death by Starvation

If you cannot find a doctor to care for you, if you don't have ready access to a provider, you don't get timely care. Untreated, your illness progresses. You suffer. If the condition is serious, you may die.

The lawyers have a saying: "Justice delayed is justice denied."[1] The doctors have their own version: "Late is always too late."

The U.S. has a critical shortage of doctors and nurses because the cancer is starving the doctors. The bureaucratic diversion described in chapter 6 is the mechanism and the bureaucracy isn't even subtle about it. ACA balances its budget on the backs of providers: The law takes $716 billion out of Medicare payments to doctors in order to defray some of the $2.6 trillion it spends on the bureaucracy.

Between 1995 and 2010, applications to U.S. medical schools fell by over 20 percent.[2] There are now over half a million unfilled nursing positions in the U.S. Provider shortages and the consequent lack of needed services can be linked directly to cutting provider reimbursements. As Robert Moffit of Heritage Foundation testified before Congress, "You cannot get more of something by paying less for it."[3]

A friend and colleague who is the Chief of a Heart Surgery Training Program shared with me a worrisome fact. There were 110 certified training positions open in U.S. cardiac surgery programs. Sixty doctors applied. Forty were graduates of U.S. medical schools. Think about what that means for people who will need heart surgery in the future. Would you want to train for nine (!) years after medical school, and be older than thirty-five before you got your first real job as a cardiac surgeon? Before you say yes, dreaming of your big salary, remember the $150,000 in student loans you will have to start paying off. I am surprised that even forty applied.

Providers are human. Like everyone else, they respond to financial incentives. If you pay them less and less, they understand that they are not valued and choose other professions. When you pay them less, you will get less *from* them and less *of* them.

> People who live in the big House White
> Proclaim health care a gov-given right.
> Then they tighten the purses,
> Starve doctors and nurses,
> And give patients a heart-stopping fright.

Death by Pressing

Though I mentioned the money first as a reason for the doctor shortage, it is less of a problem than the regulatory burden. The fact is doctors are dying by being "pressed."

"Pressing" was a form of death-by-torture devised by colonial Americans and dramatized by the great American playwright, Arthur Miller in his play, *The Crucible*. Written in 1953 during the McCarthy hysteria to "get the Reds out," Miller set his play in Massachusetts during the Salem witch trials (1692-93). His award-winning play was an allegory for the scourge of McCarthyism.

Near the end of Miller's play, Elizabeth tells John Proctor the story of Corey Gilles, who was *pressed to death*. Where the Romans crucified; the Russians staked out heretics; and the Europeans burned people alive; Americans pressed.

Pressing involved putting more and more weights on the chest of an accused until the weight of rocks made it impossible to breath. Like Jesus, the victim died of asphyxiation.

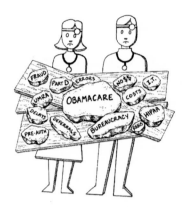

People who work in healthcare increasingly feel just like Miller's character Corey Giles. The red tape, ever-increasing complexity, incomprehensible rules and regulations, followed by more "explanatory" rules and regulations; the constantly expanding reach of Federal agencies; a dizzying array of administrative processes, organizational charts and compliance mandates: these are all "weights" being placed on care providers.

The bureaucracy keeps adding more and more weights until our health care providers cannot breathe. The weights, the BARRC, the stolen resources, they make it impossible for providers to do what you expect them to do (and what they *want* to do): Care for you.

Some people believe that money, specifically the lack of it, is the main reason why men and women are leaving the care side of the medical profession in droves. Not so! Scientific studies show that money is not the main cause of dissatisfaction among health care professionals. The primary reasons are hassle factor/bureaucratic burden and the heavy responsibility with no authority.[4]

I have talked at length about how difficult it is to practice medicine under the current huge mass of administrative rules and with the bureaucracy constantly cutting support. Both private insurers and government reduce their spending in two ways: Using administrative excuses to delay payment for care and by cutting the amount of money paid to providers and institutions. Remember, the government never cuts payments to the bureaucracy—that would be suicide for them.

When health care providers are pressed to death by the cancer's suffocating BARRC, it is really a death spiral for We The Patients.

Death By Lack of Insurance

The U.S. has an insurance-based system for the financing of health care. That means, as my next-door neighbor and insurance salesman says, "Small contributions of the many pay for the large expenses of the few."

Insurance is a betting pool where you hope you "lose" and stay a loser. The "winners" are the ones who collect. They are the people who have major illnesses needing expensive care. You put in your small bet and hope you stay healthy. In the U.S., insurance is, or used to be, the gateway to getting medical care.

Health insurance premiums are inordinately expensive. You know why: federal BARRC; internal administration of insurance companies; cost of the uninsured (the unfunded mandates); and profits. Interestingly, insurance profits, while a huge number in our minds, is only a minor factor compared to the other reasons why health insurance is so costly.

Our insurance premiums are going up. Just open your next bill and check. Some experts think that insurance premiums will double in the near future.[5] We have two choices. We can continue to pay them, or we can opt out of insurance altogether and pay the IRS fine. Either way, we're still left vulnerable if we get sick.

The math is simple. You couldn't afford health insurance before ACA, so the gate to health care service was then closed. Now with Obamacare, the cost of insurance has gone up, so the gate (to the doctor's office) is now padlocked, maybe even closed and boarded up.

And don't forget, if you do have insurance but there are no doctors, you still die, just with insurance rather than without.

Death By Budget

Say your heart is failing and you need a transplant. You don't have $250,000 in cash lying around, and your insurance won't cover the transplant. Your heart stops and you die. Or maybe your insurance does cover the transplant but only at a cheap hospital with inferior outcomes, and you still die.

You have just succumbed to death by budget.

There are numerous safety nets in place in the U.S. to prevent any person—citizen or illegal resident—from dying by lack of care due to being poor. Some of these protections work well. Many do not. Then there are those who don't use the government-provided insurance that is available to them. These people avoid going to the doctor until they are desperate and then show up in the Emergency Department (ED), often too late. Their fear of un-payable bills and lack of insurance coverage kills them.

Americans die by budget because the costs of both health care and health insurance are too high to pay.

Some might point to nations that have universal health care, and say, People there do not die *"by budget."* Even ignoring the fact that non-citizens in these nations do not get care at all without paying out of pocket, countries such as Canada and Great Britain have the same death-by-budget problem that we do.[6]

For some time, newspapers in Great Britain have been reporting cutbacks in health services such as maternity benefits and hospice care. We already know about surgeries are being delayed by putting people in the queue. Death by queueing is really a type of death by budget.

To our north, Canada also has death by budget. In 2004, a Canadian physician named Dr. Ciaran McNamee sued the Alberta Provincial government, claiming that people were dying needlessly while waiting for approved surgery. His suit cited cases going back to 1998 that demonstrated scheduling delays for operations, especially heart surgery, that were causing avoidable deaths.

Dr. McNamee attributed the fatal delays to a Canadian healthcare system that authorized care but funded too few operating rooms and insufficient nurses and doctors to perform surgeries in timely fashion. In other words, the government allocated too little money to provide the promised, needed, and medically appropriate care.

The issue came to a head in March 2011, breaking on the major Canadian TV networks. The picture clip shows all the party leaders, who are usually trading barbs, actually demanding in unison a formal inquiry.[7] The sad part is that for at least thirteen years, Canadian citizens were dying unnecessarily while waiting for authorized health care. The sadder part is that they still are.

Do not, however, instantly conclude that Canada needs to spend more money. In England and Canada, just as in the US, the problem is not too little spending on healthcare. The problem is spending on the wrong things.

Several years ago, a friend and colleague testified before our New Mexico Senate about the State healthcare budget. He had the audacity to say to the Senators, "We don't need more money in healthcare. We just need to distribute it better." (I am surprised he got out of our State Capitol, called the Roundhouse, with all body parts intact.)

I really need to pound this point home: huge amounts of money go into the healthcare the system but do not come out—that is, do not come out as health *care*. People in the commercial world call this "non-value-adding steps." You and I call it *wasting my money*. Successful businesses take great pains to eliminate this type of inefficiency. Federal governments take great pains to *add* non-value-adding steps, i.e., more bureaucracy.

In response to an article that I published on AmericanThinker.com, a Canadian posted the following comment about the administrative cost of their system. "If you think [U.S.] health care is expensive now, wait till yours is 'free.' We have 'free healthcare' here in Canada. It costs 60 cents of every federal tax dollar I pay."[6]

Lest you think such problems that occur with universal health care won't happen here, take a look at Massachusetts. I've already pointed out that women in the Bay State with abdominal pain have to wait more than forty days to see a doctor. That's because the Massachusetts healthcare system, called Commonwealth Care, was based on the British system and was also used as a model for ACA. Does it make you feel any better or safer when you or your wife, in pain, has to wait six weeks to find out whether she has cancer, ulcers, a pelvic infection, or gas? Is that what you call the "prompt access to high quality care" we were promised?

Even before implementation of ACA, fifty-seven percent of internists and forty-six percent of family practice doctors in Massachusetts said they could not accept government-financed patients. Now with ACA's further reduced reimbursement schedules, those numbers are going up. Doctors' costs per patient are greater than what they are being paid by the government. So, when doctors accept new Obmacare patients, they simply accelerate their trip to bankruptcy court and out of medical practice.

Massachusetts is not an isolated case. In 1993, the State of Maine implemented what authors Tarren Bragdon and Joel Allumbaugh dubbed "Obamacare Lite."[8] In 2011, Maine had to reverse its decision. The costs of insurance premiums had gone up, not down. The State had provided hundreds of millions of dollars in subsidies and even so, the number of uninsured Maine residents went *up*. The reason I mention this is simple: many of us knew what was coming with Obamacare and President Obama should have known too. (Maybe he did?!)

The money for ACA goes to the government from us, directly via taxes and penalties, or indirectly through insurance companies. The government then pays the healthcare bureaucracy first, which is literally the government paying itself. That is why they always cut our service and never cut their own pay. What little is left is used for patient care.

Always remember the cancer's mantra: ***Feed the bureaucracy by cutting the service.***

Some people say health care is our right. They quote the second paragraph of the U.S. Declaration of Independence as their proof: "We hold these truths to be self-evident, that all men are created equal, that they are endowed by their Creator with certain unalienable Rights, that among these are Life, Liberty and the pursuit of Happiness." It might seem logical that a right to "Life" would mean a right to health care. If someone does not care for our health, we won't have it for long.

What is left after the bureaucracy takes the first and biggest piece of the pie doesn't give us the care we need. It seems that the bureaucracy's "right" to feed comes before our right to live. Don't you find this ... alarming? Personally, I would use the word frightening.

Dr. Seuss books were a staple in our home when our children were growing up. My wife had met the author—Ted Geisel—and described him as an exceedingly caring person who was quite shy not only with adults but even with children. The following online, unattributed poem was written in Dr. Seuss' style but not by him. I suspect that Ted Geisel would have liked it:

> I do not like this Uncle Sam,
>> Especially not his health care scam.
> I do not like Washington dirty crooks,
>> Or how they lie and cook the books.
> I do not like when Congress steals.
>> I do not like their secret deals.
> I do not like ex-speaker Nan,
>> I do not like her false "Yes WE Can."
> I do not like their spending spree.
>> I'm smart. I know that nothing's free.
> I do not like their smug replies,
>> When I complain about their lies.
> I do not like their kind of hope.
>> I do not like it. Nope, nope, nope!

Paul Farmer is an MD and noted anthropologist. Speaking about the right to health care with his physician hat on, he said, "I can argue that no one should have to die of a disease that is treatable."

I hope the irony is not lost on you. It does seem to elude those who advocate government control of healthcare. If Congressional allocations determine what care you get or don't get, then you will die by budget, despite having a treatable illness. Dr. Farmer would call this unconscionable and unethical. I would agree, which is why I had to quit medical practice after ACA became law.

Death By "Either/Or"

This type of demise is really an extension of death by budget, but you have to understand how non-healthcare governmental agencies and activities—important ones like our military and our schools—are being affected by the "either/or" situation that an ever expanding healthcare bureaucracy intentionally creates.

Let's look at the military first. In 2009, Defense Secretary Robert Gates testified before Congress that healthcare costs were "eating the [Defense] Department alive." He made the telling comparison that the Pentagon pays just about as much for fighter aircraft and high-tech weapons as it does to the healthcare system for ten million active duty personnel, retirees, reservists, and their families.

The average American civilian family of four pays $6,328 per year for a private health insurance.[9] Those who are covered by TRICARE—the military's health care insurance system—pay the same as they did eleven years ago: $230 per year for an individual and $460 for a family.[10]

I have already pointed out the money the Department of Defense (DoD) pays for healthcare. The revenue paid to the DoD by military families accounts for less than 10 percent (in reality closer to 1 percent) of what the DoD spends on healthcare. That difference must come out of the military budget.[11]

I'm not saying that military families shouldn't have health insurance. What I am pointing out is that there is a sinister either/or at work. Either our soldiers will have enough equipment to protect themselves, or their families will have their health costs fully paid. In other words, spending on healthcare is putting our soldiers' lives at risk.

Either/Or also endangers our children.

Atul Gawande is a Harvard surgeon and frequent contributor to *The New Yorker* on healthcare issues. He wrote about a conversation he had with the Superintendent of his own children's school.

> Dr. Gawande: "Superintendent, I'm so glad I ran in to you."
>
> Superintendent (defensively stepping back): "Are you going to complain, too?"
>
> Dr. Gawande: "I don't know about what others have said but I am worried about what is happening in my children's classes. Has art totally been cut out of the curriculum? And the student/teacher ratios seem to be

going up, with some classes even thirty-to-one. Isn't this bad for the children?"

Superintendent: "You think I don't know it?! What do you think I spend most of my time on? Curriculum improvements? Test scores? Hiring teachers? Building new classrooms? Nope. The issue that consumes most of my time is ... healthcare costs."

The Superintendent paused, thought for a moment, and then continued. "City tax revenue hasn't gone up. Student enrollment has. Allocations are dropping, while the costs keep going up. This year alone, the cost of teacher health care benefits has increased 9 percent. So I have more students, less money, and more costs. What can I do?"

Dr. Gawande wanted to give him a reason for hope, but he couldn't. He walked away with his head down.[12]

The Boston school Superintendent and Defense Secretary Gates have the same "either/or" conundrum because of overspending by Congress on the U.S. healthcare system. Such spending is crowding out other, worthy national expenditures, such as Education, Military, and Infrastructure maintenance and upgrading.

Death by either/or hurts everyone and everything.

Death By Panel

The mere mention of the phrase "Death Panel" seems to stop all rational discussion. A "death panel" is a group of bureaucrats who decide whether or not certain types of illnesses would be deemed "treatable" and worth the cost of government money.

The uproar started when Sarah Palin charged on Facebook that government-run healthcare would create these "death panels." Some argued that her accusation was ludicrous and provided unequivocal proof that she will make up any outrageous statement just to get press coverage. Others see her claim as absolutely true, without question.

As with all matters like this, it's up to you to examine the facts and make up your own mind.

Do Death Panels exist? Might they be real? Could you or I have to face one?

The *real* Death Panels will never face an actual live human being.

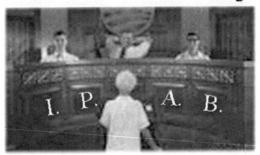

Part of the confusion is a basic misunderstanding about what "death panels" are. They are not a panel of "Big Brothers" that decides whether or not an individual should receive care. "Death panels" do not judge whether or not an individual lives or dies. Those kinds of panels are actually called Star Chambers. Hundreds of years ago, Princes would decide life or death for a specific peasant or minor noble. Thousands of years ago, in the Roman Coliseum, the audience would put thumbs up (for life) or down (for death) for a single person in the arena.

A "Death Panel" is more ... bureaucratic. These are committees that make medical decisions about groups of people and types of illnesses, not about specific individuals. In chapter 7, I talked about the "Independent Payment Advisory Board" or IPAB in the section on the myth of "single payer is good for you." IPAB may sound innocuous, but it makes your life-or-death decisions. The government, through the ACA's IPAB, makes health policy decisions for the general population based *not* on whether a treatment works on you, but whether or not that treatment is "cost effective," meaning whether it fits within the budget.

Baby S. was born early, ten weeks before he was due. He weighed less than two pounds. Because he was born with a hole in his diaphragm, his left lung was very under-developed. The baby spent the next five months in the neonatal intensive care unit, much of it on a ventilator (mechanical breathing machine). He required two major surgeries, one-on-one nursing for months, and multiple, diverse expensive medications. At discharge, the hospital bill was $994,876.44. At two years of age, Baby S. is a perfectly normal child as far as we can tell. Was his treatment "cost effective"?

When a Death Panel declares some medical treatment "Not cost-effective," that says nothing about whether the therapy will work to save you or your child. "Not cost-effective" means that the treatment is considered too costly for what the budget has allocated. That is the rationale behind age limits for various procedures, including many treatments that do work but are expensive.

To give you an example of how these panels work: a few years ago, the British NHS declared kidney dialysis (mechanical cleansing of the blood) after age fifty-five, open-heart surgery after sixty-five, and all hospice care as "Not cost-effective." Though the treatments are effective and would likely work for you or your parent, they are not available in Great Britain under their National Health Service. Simply put, if you need dialysis to survive, too bad. You will die by Death Panel.

The real question surrounding the issue of "death panels" is whether the patient is in control of his or her personal medical decisions (preferably with a doctor's advice), or is someone else in control: an insurance rep or Medicare Director, or a group of individuals such as an expert panel, a Congressional, subcommittee or advisory board.

We know that ultimately we are responsible for our health, and therefore we should be in control of its care. We are not (in control) and the evidence proves it.

For instance, did you know that ACA reduces the amount you can contribute to an HSA (Health Savings Account) to $2,500? I bet you didn't. HSA's are one of the few ways that patients might re-assert control of their own health care spending. So why would the federal government want to cut HSA's? Answer: to reduce our control of our dollars so we will be more dependent on its bureaucracy.

A few months ago, I was one of three speakers on a public forum about healthcare. Sitting next to me at the head table was a man who was a doctor-lawyer: he had both an MD degree and a JD (Doctor of Jurisprudence). He was both an experienced (internal medicine) physician and world-renown legal expert on medical ethics. He gave his speech from a wheelchair. In fact, it was astonishing that he came to New Mexico from his home in Texas. He had kidney failure, was on dialysis, and was waiting for a match to get a kidney transplant.

I could not help staring at him, thinking to myself: This great contributor to our world, this "beautiful mind" would be lost if he lived in England.[13] Given his age and condition, the British NHS would decree his death—by panel decision.

Again, the comparisons between our ACA and Britain's NHS abound. Where the NHS has its NICE (National Institute for Clinical Excellence), ACA has IPAB (Independent payment Advisory Board). NICE and IPAB do the same thing. They say what the national budget can afford. What the budget allocation does not cover is deemed Not Cost Effective. Call it what you will—I call this death by panel.

The Liverpool Care Protocol

Believe it or not, there is something even worse than death panels. What is described above is the government—through NICE or IPAB— allowing you to die *passively*. Given bureaucracy's insatiable greed, it's not that far down a slippery slope to have it actively *killing* you.

I can just hear you thinking, "Deane has gone over the edge. He's crazy! My government would never, ever do that to me!"

WAIT!! Before you dismiss me as a complete lunatic, let me show you why I am afraid, and why you should be too.

The NHS has started to offer financial incentives to British providers and hospitals if they enroll critically ill patients in the LCP (Liverpool Care Protocol). Once enrolled, all complex (read expensive), treatments are withheld from the patients. So is nutrition. The patient is sedated and quietly killed, even when they might be saved.[14]

Remember in chapter 7 where I talked about the Florida sanity hearings and how many were declared insane because the psychiatrist made more money? Ask yourself how many people would be killed rather than saved because of the financial incentives in LCP? I shudder to think.

The LCP is state-encouraged euthanasia. Under the guise of allowing "patients to die in peace," the NHS is actively killing them, just like the Nazis did. This time those who die by state decree will be the *expensives*—old and ill—rather than the politically undesirable.

You can try to sugar coat it and call LCP a "care" program. But, to any doctor who ever read, much less swore, the Hippocratic Oath—to anyone who understands the law— facilitating the end of someone's life against their will is called murder.[15]

Since ACA was modeled after the NHS, you know that what England does today will come to this side of the Atlantic tomorrow. If you think, "My government will never ever do that to me," perhaps you need to think again.

Death By Instant Gratification

There's another force at work in healthcare, and it's something that none of us want to confront. If we're sick, we expect to take our pill, get better, and be done with it. We also have the same mentality with budgets: most national governments, including the U.S., focus on short-term financials, specifically next year's spending. They pay no attention to the long-term results, either for our money or for our health. As a result, they spend more than they should and more than they need to.

Many years ago, I was part of a panel discussion at the American Academy of Pediatrics Annual Meeting about medical economics. They wanted me to discuss the finances, not the medicine, of what pediatric cardiologists like me did—caring for children with congenital heart disease. My work was chosen because the costs of what we do in pediatric cardiology are so high. The other panelists were an insurance agent, a hospital Chief Financial Officer, and a health care economist (self-styled).

We spent some time explaining to the audience what each person did and why the costs were so high. Then the following dialogue took place:

Me: So, the last child we repaired with transposition of the great arteries generated a bill of $186,285 for his hospital stay—from the time he was born until he was discharged at sixteen days of age.

Economist: Are you saying the hospital bill was around $11,000 per day?

Me: Yep, your math sounds right.

Economist: Don't you think that is exorbitant?

Me: Exorbitant? No. A huge bill, yes.

Economist: Aren't you embarrassed expecting the insurance company to pay an eighth of a million dollars for a two-week hospital stay? Isn't that, well, ridiculous? What will the public think?

Me: I can tell you for a fact that the parents were overjoyed. They saw their baby born cyanotic (blue from lack of oxygen) and took home a smiling, pink baby.

Economist: Yes, that's lovely and heart-warming. But we are here to talk about money. So, please justify to all of us a bill of almost two hundred thousand dollars.

Me: Let's say you were an investor. Would you pay $186,285 for an investment that would pay for over $2 million?

Economist: Of course I would. That is more than a ten-fold return on my money. Where can I get one?

Me: You just got one. I read somewhere that over the course of a working lifetime, the average U.S. worker generates about $2.8 million more than the costs to educate and train him or her. So, assuming the child with repaired transposition lives a normal lifespan, you just spent a hundred and eighty-five thousand to get back over two million.

Economist: Yes, but, but …

Me: But what? Is there something wrong with my math?

*Economist: No, not the math, the time frame. You are making me spend a hundred and eighty-five thousand dollars <u>today</u> and expecting me to wait more than **fifty years** for the pay-off! That's not what I want.*

Me: Precisely, yes, exactly! That may not be what you want as an investor, but that is exactly what people want from our healthcare system. They want to spend now and expect the pay-off to continue over decades, over a lifetime in fact.

Everyone from the President to the average person-in-the-street seems to have tunnel vision when it comes to healthcare. They focus exclusively on the *now*. How much will it cost today? Will I be able to go back to work tomorrow? How much can I cut from next month's projected spending? How will today's decisions affect the next election cycle? (Two years is the longest time horizon that politicians have.)

Failure to include the *long-term, desired benefits* in any calculation produces a bad decision. I call this death by instant gratification. If all you consider is how to cut next month's spending, the cheapest solution to any major illness is death! Thirty years ago, I made a picture to demonstrate this point. It showed a bullet and called it "The cheapest solution to congenital heart disease." My wife made me promise never to use it in a public talk, and I haven't. I am just giving you the idea of the image.

Let's move from the ludicrous to the practical. Say you want to buy a car. As a smart and experienced shopper, what would do you?

First, you would check your bank account to see how much money you can spend. (Note that your first act is the one thing that the federal government *never* does at all!) Then you would probably go to the Internet to start shopping. You would compare makes and models, look at features like miles-per-gallon and maintenance schedules, and certainly determine *all* costs. This includes initial payment, ongoing expenses such as gas, monthly loan payments, and maintenance. You look at the design of the various models, from different angles, on your computer screen. (No need to go to the showroom unless you want to test-drive the car.)

You consider alternatives such using public transportation rather than buying a car. You look up reported problems and resale value in Consumer reports. Now you are ready to calculate a long-term cost-to-benefit ratio (the benefit you get for the price you pay). You want something that's going to last but isn't going to cost you too much money.

Do you do the same thing when you purchase health insurance? Not a chance. As a patient, you have no access to the same type of information that you demand when buying an automobile. And what is more important to you: Your car or living a long, healthy life? We don't even think about a cost-to-benefit ratio about our lives. We'll do pretty much anything to survive, but we want everything to happen *now*. We don't think about twenty, thirty, or fifty years into the future.

For the public as well as the insurance carriers, all they see is the *now*. Such thinking produces death while seeking instant gratification because they want and expect everything to be taken care of right now instead of looking at the long-term.

This has some pretty severe consequences: Do you know health-care's definition of successful heart surgery? "Success" is either being discharged alive from the hospital, or living more than thirty days after operation. That's it. If you are still having chest pain; if you cannot return to work; if you still cannot climb a flight of stairs, even if you are still in ICU on day thirty-one or die after hospital discharge, you are nonetheless listed in the "successful surgery" column. For healthcare, long-term is not measured and therefore does not exist.

Death By Bleeding

Back in the dark ages, doctors used to bleed patients, literally. People thought that the blood contained the disease so getting rid of it would cure you. Some historians argue that George Washington's doctor bled him to death accidentally while *treating* a throat infection.[16] Bleeding patients was an accepted medical practice in those days to remove "evil humors."

In healthcare terms, you could say that the government appropriates, diverts, pilfers, siphons, steals, or takes the funds needed for health care without permission. Being a doctor, I prefer medical, anatomic, lurid, (okay gory) terminology. I say that we are being bled to death by a parasite, a leech, a vampire—the cancer of greed, particularly of the bureaucratic variety.

This is happening to all of us except those favored few who were given exemptions from ACA. In chapters six and seven, you saw how individual citizens are being bled dry by insurance premiums, health care costs, as well as ACA taxes and penalties.

The bureaucracy is also sucking the providers dry. Recall that ACA law cuts $716 billion dollars from Medicare payments to doctors.

But the one most damaged by the bureaucratic bloodsucking is our nation.

How much money is being consumed (how much blood is being sucked out of us) by the healthcare system? First, note that spending on healthcare is the largest line item on the entire U.S. budget, larger than defense or social security. Gross Domestic Product (GDP) is a common indicator of how well a country is doing economically. A comparison of healthcare spending with GDP is informative. In 1960 the U.S. spent five percent of GDP on our healthcare system. By 2011, healthcare had consumed 17.9 percent of GDP, which translated to $2.7 trillion. Analysts say we are heading for twenty percent.[17] You might want to re-look at graphic in chapter 2 that showed what a trillion dollars looks like.

To put this amount of money—blood as it were—in perspective, the U.S. "bled" more for healthcare than any nation on earth *produced* as their total GDP with only four exceptions: China, India, Japan, and Germany. Think about it this way. We spent more on our healthcare system in one year than all the money produced by countries such as Russia, Brazil, Great Britain, or France.

Who is the bloodsucker? A greedy cancer. However, there is a big difference between how much "blood" corporate greed takes and the amount that bureaucratic cancer sucks out of us. The corporate fat cats take their profits in the millions, but the bureaucrats bleed us in the trillions.

Last year alone, you and I "bled" $2,700,000,000,000 (2.7 trillion dollars) for our healthcare system. Forty percent of that—$1,000,000,000,000 (one trillion) —went to bureaucrats instead of to nurses and doctors. That's a *lot* of ... blood (money.)

Remember that maze-like organizational chart I showed you in chapter 7 on ACA's overwhelmingly complex organization structure? Well, you and I pay for all of it. Our blood feeds all those lines of connection, those boxes, circles, oblongs, rhomboids, and stars, each of which represents dozens-to-thousands of bureaucrats. This chart represents trillions of our dollars taken, sucked out of our wallets, and then diverted from health *care* to support the healthcare bureaucracy.

Over its first ten years (2010-2020), ACA will bleed us to the tune of anywhere between $1.7 trillion to $2.6 trillion in additional, new spending.[18] What will ACA do with all that money? Why, feed the bureaucracy of course. You didn't think we would actually get more health *care*, did you?

Dollar Inefficiency Is Killing Us

You know what dollar efficiency means from chapter 6: The money that goes in to a process, system, or organization, which produces desired outcomes. Examples of desired outcomes could be building a product for a consumer or providing a service to a client, or restoring health to a patient.

A successful auto manufacturer sells lots of cars. He builds the best cars he can for his market and tries to be dollar-efficient to keep his costs down while using the dollars to add value. That means spending most of his money on the car, and as little as possible on administration and bureaucracy overhead. The car itself offers value to the customer. Money spent on BARRC does not: it is wasteful, non-value-adding, and is definitely dollar inefficient.

If our healthcare system were dollar-efficient, we would see the bulk of our money paying for provider services, hospital care, medications, and durable goods like scalpels, wheelchairs, and pacemakers. When healthcare spends forty percent of its money (our blood) on the bureaucracy, especially the regulatory machine, it is extremely dollar *inefficient*. And when it has to take money from health care *service* to grow the healthcare *bureaucracy*, it is worse than inefficient. It is killing us.

The blood sucking is killing us three times over. First, we die from lack of blood, literally, in our bodies. Our hearts have nothing to circulate around, and we die.

Second, we die from lack of care. The blood/money taken from us that was supposed to support our care providers is diverted from the providers to the bureaucrats. Without nurses and doctors, who will care for us? Are you comfortable with Nancy Pelosi making your diagnosis, Barack Obama wielding the scalpel, and Harry Reid as your ICU nurse?

Finally, our blood (our money)—desperately needed to "feed" other activities like education, defense, infrastructure, and social services—is being consumed by the bureaucratic cancer. The blood being consumed by the bureaucratic cancer is being taken from these other sorely needed activities just as it is stolen from caregivers.

On November 19, 1863, at the dedication of the Soldiers' National Cemetery, President Abraham Lincoln gave his famous Gettysburg Address. He reminded us that we were fighting for no less than the soul of our nation, a nation that claimed to have a "government of the people, by the people, [and] for the people." It wouldn't have sounded right if he had said a "government of the politicians, by the regulators, and for the bureaucrats." In Lincoln's worst nightmare, I doubt that he ever dreamt that our "government of the people, by the people and for the people" could "perish from the earth," because it was bled to death by the cancer of bureaucratic greed.

Our dreams are turned to nightmares. Our usual allies apparently are our enemies. Our ultimate ally is not behaving the way we think an ally should and we now know why: Cancer.

The cancer in the federal bureaucracy—through its BARRC—is devouring us, bite by bite, and its bite appears to be lethal.

President Obama promised to save us. Is his namesake reform of our healthcare system—Obamacare—our savior or something else, more sinister?

NINE

The ACA Scorecard

We know that our healthcare system is sick. We now know why it is so ill and that the sickness it has could be fatal. A treatment plan for sick patient Healthcare, called ACA, has been started against the wishes of a majority of Americans. Is Obamacare working? Is it delivering on its promises? We now have hard evidence.

Michael Cerpok is one of six children born to a schoolteacher. He dropped out of high school to start work at age seventeen. With nothing but hard work over nearly three decades, he now owns two businesses. He is an American success story, yet he may not be able to afford health insurance.[1]

"I've worked hard because I've had to, and I've had to, because cancer runs in my family," said Cerpok, who picked his health insurance based on that family history. His monthly premium was just about half of his monthly take-home pay.

Back in 2006, he found out he had an incurable form of leukemia that can be controlled but not cured. He requires expensive ongoing treatments to stay alive. In 2012, his treatment bill was more than $350,000. But because of his pre-ACA insurance, his out-of-pocket was only $4,500 a year.

That changed when Michael's insurance carrier sent a letter saying he would be dropped from coverage. Why? Because Obamacare regulations require the carrier to offer "better" insurance as promised by the President. That insurance is just a *liii*ttle more expensive.

"It [ACA] doesn't mean I can't go see my current doctor, but my $4,500 out-of-pocket, is going to turn into a minimum of $26,000 out-of-pocket to see the doctor that I've been seeing the last seven years," he said.

In fact, Michael can't continue to see the doctor he has been seeing for seven years, because the physician just took early retirement, in response to ACA.

You know from the previous nine chapters how sick patient Healthcare has been for decades and how it was hurting both We The Patients and our country. "Doctor" Obama proposed a treatment plan called ACA. Some of us worried about the results. Many of those concerns are offered in the prior chapters. However, those fears were purely theoretical.

When the first edition of this book was published in 2013, Obamacare had been law of the land for three years but had not yet been implemented. ACA took effect in January 2014. Therefore, now (2015), we can look at evidence of what the ACA has done, rather than depend on promises, estimates, and predictions.

Has the ACA produced the outcomes that we were promised? Has Obamacare lived up to its hype? What does the evidence tell us?

The Promises of ACA

Here is the list of assurances that President Obama gave the American people about what his namesake law would accomplish for us:

- Bend down the U.S. healthcare spending curve: Reduce national spending
- Make health care affordable for all
- Insure all Americans
- Provide "all the care that Americans deserve"
- "If you like your doctor, you can keep your doctor."
- "If you like your insurance plan, you can keep your insurance plan."

Now let's compare the above assurances with the evidence-of-effect—the proof of what Obamacare has actually done to us or for us.

Reduce National Spending

Many people forget the reason the president started his self-styled reform of healthcare. It wasn't the uninsured or substandard (his term) insurance. It was the amount the U.S. was spending on our healthcare system, an amount our nation cannot afford.

In 1970, the U.S. was spending roughly the same amount as other developed nations on healthcare. Over the next four decades, everyone increased their spending on health care in part because of the marvelous but expensive technological advances.

In 1994, one of my closest friends named Larry was saved by a stent placed to open a narrowing in his coronary artery. The charge was $35,000. In 1970, Larry could not have had the procedure because stents did not exist. Larry would just have died but we would not have spent $35,000.

In 1970, when I was training in Pediatrics, every child with leukemia died. Their deaths "saved" us the large expenses of chemotherapy.

Medical miracles notwithstanding, the graph below shows what has happened. All those technological miracles were available in all the countries displayed just like the U.S. Yet, we spend twice what everyone else is spending.[2] Therefore, our over-spending is not due to the expense of modern technologies.

Healthcare Spending, by Country

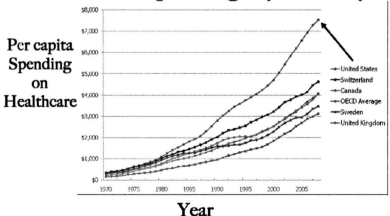

Per capita Spending on Healthcare

Year

The first estimate for the cost of ACA was $900 billion. Then it was $1.1 trillion, then $1.7 trillion, and the current best guess is over $2.6 trillion.[3] The difference between the first estimate and the best one for the cost of Obamacare is equal to the total GDP of India. An error of this magnitude could send our nation into bankruptcy court.

We have good reasons to worry about the reliability of Washington cost estimates. In chapter 5, I pointed out that when Congress passed the Medicare Act in 1964, they did so based on what they thought was a reliable and affordable cost prediction over twenty-five years. In 1990, with twenty-five years of hard data, the CBO uncovered the true cost for—what was actually spent on—Medicare and compared that to the original estimate in 1965. The government under-estimated the cost by 854 percent. If they underestimate the actual cost of the ACA by the same amount, Obamacare would cost more than $26 trillion.[4] That amount of money is fifty percent more than the gross domestic product ($17.7 trillion) of the entire United States!

If you look at the U.S. spending as a percentage of GDP, the numbers are even more frightening. In 1970, we spent 7 percent of our GDP on healthcare. In 2012, that number was 18 percent! And that was *before* implementation of Obamacare. If we add the cost of ACA's new spending ($2.7 trillion), healthcare will easily consume well over 20 percent of GDP by 2020.

U.S. spending on healthcare is clearly growing at a rate we cannot sustain. If we keep it up, we will either go bankrupt; have our bridges all fall down, or send our troops into battle without bullets. The president was quite right in 2008 when he said we needed to reduce our healthcare spending. Did his signature plan do that?

Table I: Effect Of Obamacare On Healthcare Spending		
Year	Est. Cost of Obamacare ($$)	Effect on National Spending
2010	$0.9 tr	↑
2011	$1.1 tr	↑↑
2012	$1.7 tr	⇑
2013	$2.1 tr	⇑↑
2015	$2.7 tr	⇑⇑
tr.=trillion. ↑ = increase; = ⇑↑ moderate increase; ⇑⇑ = large increase.		

Clearly, Obamacare *increases* U.S. spending on healthcare even though the president promised that his healthcare "reform" would *decrease* spending.

ACA is having the opposite effect on national spending from what we expected.

In case you did not notice, the full effects of Obamacare will hit us in 2017, when Mr. Obama is no longer in the White House. He can then blame his successor and a Republican Congress.

If you have children or grandchildren, you should be very worried for them. Every generation of parents has wanted their children to have better lives than they had. We all feel that way, no exceptions. So, what happens when my two grandsons—at this time ages eight and five—have to pay back the trillions that the ACA is spending now? How will forcing our massive debt on my grandsons give them a better life?

I suspect you begin to see that I am not just worried. I am angry. Leaders are expected to keep their promises.

Is Health Care Now Affordable?

Next on our list of Obamacare promises is affordable health care. After all, that *is* the law's name. Does ACA deliver affordable health care to the American people? Actually, that promise became meaningless shortly after ACA was signed into law in March 2010.

In April 2010, President Obama qualified his intentions saying that his namesake Act was aimed at health *insurance* not health *care*. He continued to champion the appellation Obamacare, though by his own admission it might be more accurately called "Obama-Insurance."

Did the president deliver on his downgraded promise to provide all Americans with affordable health insurance?

"Obama thinks that he is making insurance affordable," wrote one reader to the *Mobile Press Register* in Alabama. "I just got a letter from my Blue Cross Blue Shield that if I want to keep their insurance it's going to cost me $300 more a month. I already pay $300 a month now and they're wanting right at $600 a month for this Affordable Care Act."

Why did a middle-class Texas couple receive a registered letter from their insurance carrier, Humana, informing them of a 539 percent rate increase on a policy they had had and liked for years? That policy was cancelled because it was not compliant with ACA rules. The cost for their policy increased from $212.10 per month to $1,356.60 per month. The couple is in good health with a combined income of less than $70,000, in other words, a middle-class family. For them, Obamacare turned the affordable into the unaffordable.

Cindy Vinson and Tom Waschura are big believers in the Affordable Care Act, or they were. They vote independent and are proud to say they helped elect and re-elect President Barack Obama. Like many other Bay Area residents who pay for their own medical insurance, both were floored last week when they opened their latest insurance bills. Their policies were replaced with more expensive plans that conform to all the requirements of Obama's new health care law. Vinson, of San Jose, will pay $1,800 more a year for an individual policy. Waschura, of Portola Valley, will cough up almost $10,000 more a year to insure his family of four.

It was interesting and quite ironic when a self-identified liberal blogger posted his personal ACA history.[1] "My wife and I just got our updates from Kaiser telling us what our 2014 rates will be. Her monthly was $168 and mine had been $150. We have a high deductible. We are generally healthy people who don't go to the doctor often. I barely ever go. The insurance is in case of a major catastrophe. Well, now, because of Obamacare, my wife's rate is going to $302 per month and mine is jumping to $284 per month. I am canceling insurance for us and I am not paying any f*cking penalty. What the hell kind of reform is this?"

Ashley Dionne, though a graduate of The University of Michigan, the only job she could find was as a part-time gym instructor—thirty-two hours a week for eight dollars an hour. Ashley has asthma, ulcers, and mild cerebral palsy.[5]

Ashley wrote that, "Obamacare took my monthly rate from $75 a month for full coverage on my Young Adult Plan, to $319 a month … after $6,000 in deductibles, of course. Liberals claimed this law would help the poor. I am the poor, the working poor, and I can't afford to support myself, let alone older generations and people not willing to work at all. This law has raped my future. It will keep me and kids my age from having a future at all. This is the real face of Obamacare and it isn't pretty."

Individuals are finding Obamacare is less affordable, not more. What about small businesses—the foundation of the American economic enterprise? Here is what Obamacare did directly to one business as reported in the *Zero Hedge Reader*.[6]

"My company, based in California, employs 600. We used to insure about 250 of our employees. The rest opted out. The company paid 50% of their premiums for about $750,000/yr. Under Obamacare, none can opt out without penalty, and the rates are double or triple, depending upon the plan. Our 750k for 250 employees is going to cost $2 million per year for 600 employees.

"By mandate, we have to pay 91.5% of the premium or more up from the 50% we used to pay.

"Our employees' share of the premium goes from $7/week for the cheapest plan to $30/week. 95% of my employees were on that plan. Remember, we used to pay 50% now we pay 91.5% and the premiums still go up that much!! The cheapest plan now has a deductible of $6350! Before it was $150. Employees making $9 to $10/hour, have to pay $30/week and have a $6350 deductible!!! What!!!!

"They can't afford that to be sure. Obamacare will kill their desire to seek medical care. Paying more money and getting less care: how does that help people?"

In 2013, Merrill and Litow predicted sharp rises for out-of-pocket mandated spending on health insurance, warning the American people of premium "sticker shock."[7] Their predictions came painfully true with average increases in the cost of insurance ranging from a low of 23 percent up to as much as 73 percent. Remember, these are increases over what we couldn't afford before Obamacare.[8]

Millions of policies were canceled.[9] Several insurance carriers simply stopped offering health insurance and exited the market entirely.[10] If Washington keeps tacking on costs to private insurers, soon they will all be gone, leaving only the government. Economist Jeffrey Pfeffer warned this might happen, writing in *Fortune* (2014) that, "health insurance companies are doomed."

Reporting the facts about Obamacare's implementation is why I called this book a "Post-Obamacare Edition." The evidence continues to pile up that health insurance is less affordable, not more. This is a direct consequence of the "Affordable Care Act." When queried on the increase costs Americans must pay, the president responded that we should be happy because we are getting "better" insurance. (Of course, better is defined by Washington, not us.) Maybe he should have called his healthcare "reform" the "Better But Less Affordable Insurance Act?"

Ask the Proctors of San Francisco if they think that is a good name. Before Obamacare was implemented, they had insurance through Kaiser Permanente that they liked. Kaiser had to discontinue that plan because it was not ACA compliant. The new "better" plan includes maternity benefits, healthy child visits, and coverage for dependents up to age twenty-six. The Proctors are in their sixties, so they are not planning on having more children. Their one son is thirty-one years old. The cheapest "better" insurance will cost them over $15,000 per year, which represents 25 percent of their entire, after tax, income. They would probably say the best name for ACA insurance is "Stuff We Don't Want At A Price We Can't Possibly Afford".

Things are likely to get worse. Shortly before this book went to press, a *Wall Street Journal* front page headline (May 22, 2015) read, "Health insurers seek big increases." Reporter Louise Radnofsky wrote that the cost of health insurance premiums will surge again, this time an additional 25 percent in Oregon to 52 percent in my home state of New Mexico in 2016. The carriers are experiencing a cost explosion due to Obamacare. They either pass on the increased medical and regulatory expenses to the consumer—that's you and me—or stop selling health insurance.

If you did not start this chapter upset about what Obamacare has done to you, I bet you are disturbed now, maybe getting as angry as I am.

Insure All Americans

Another of President Obama's promises was to insure all Americans. How did that work out?

Edie Littlefield Sundby is someone you will never see at a media event with the President. He wrote the following:[6]

"My grievance is not political; all my energies are directed to enjoying life and staying alive, and I have no time for politics. For almost seven years I have fought and survived stage-4 gallbladder cancer, with a five-year survival rate of less than 2% after diagnosis. I am a determined fighter and extremely lucky. But this luck may have just run out: My affordable, lifesaving medical insurance policy has been canceled effective Dec. 31, 2013. My choice is to get coverage through the government health exchange and lose access to my cancer doctors, or pay much more for insurance outside the exchange (the quotes average 40% to 50% more) for the privilege of starting over with an unfamiliar insurance company and impaired benefits."

Well over seven million Americans lost the insurance that they liked because of Obamacare. Washington estimates that ten million people[11] gained insurance through the ACA, almost all through Medicaid expansion where insurance is "free" to the recipients. The net gain is roughly 2.5 million newly insured Americans, or a two percent reduction in the uninsured.

ACA costs $2.6 trillion. That means *Obamacare will spend $10,400,000 for each and every newly insured person.* I bet you are angry now!

And why are some exempt? Seriously, if Obamacare is good for everyone, per President Obama, why would anyone want to be exempt?

Exceptions, Waivers, and Exemptions

The dry cleaning establishment my wife and I use regularly is owned and operated by Susanna and Roberto. They are illegal residents who have been here for sixteen years and have been trying to become legal for most of that entire time. An impenetrable system plus constant rule changes have left them illegal despite their best efforts.

Recently, Roberto was picked up in a random sweep while visiting a friend in Arizona. He was held in a detention center for over two months waiting for a hearing that would presumably deport him. Through the efforts of many citizens here in New Mexico along with his wife and seven children, the Arizona judge released Roberto; gave him a green card; and said that he and his family were, "precisely the kind of people we want here in the U.S."

Susanna and Roberto have twelve employees, probably all here illegally. (I don't ask questions when I don't want to hear the answers.) They all pay taxes. For their family, their employees and their employees' families, private insurance is unaffordable, and government insurance is unavailable, by law. So, they get no routine care. If they have an emergency, you know where they have to go. You also know who will pay the bill.

Every administration since EMTALA was passed in 1986 (see chapter 5) has neatly sidestepped the conundrum that Congress created called the "unfunded mandate". Illegal residents are forbidden to obtain government-supported health insurance, yet hospitals are required to provide all their care even though there is no payment source.

ACA continues this "policy" of having no coherent policy. Undocumented residents are denied insurance and yet they get care without insurance, while the rest of us are required to buy insurance and penalized if we don't.

How should undocumented residents be treated by the U.S. healthcare system? Should they be excluded from the system entirely, as universal health care systems do in Germany and Great Britain? Should illegals continue in limbo as they are now? How is that fair?

If having everyone insured is good for both individuals and for our nation, why are illegals excluded? For that matter, if having ACA insurance is good for people, why are there thousands of exemptions? I have talked about those who are exempt in previous chapters and asked the question, if ACA is "good for everyone," then why would anyone want an exemption? Plenty of people. Here's a small sampling of the more than *fourteen hundred* ACA exemptions:

Selected exemptions from Obamacare mandates	
Allied Building Inspectors IUOE Local 211	Jakov P. Dulcich & Sons
Bowman Sheet Metal Heating & A/C	JLG Harvesting, Inc.
Carey Johnson Oil Co, Inc	MO-Kan Teamsters and Welfare Fund
Cement Masons' Local No. 502	North States Industries Inc*
City of Olathe, Kansas	Roofers Local 8 Insurance & Trust Fund
Congress itself and its staff	SCC Healthcare Group, LLP
Employer-Teamsters Local Nos. 175 & 505	Sieben Polk Law Firm
GC Harvesting, Inc.	Taylor Farms
Indiana Area UFCW Union Locals and Retail Food Employers' Health and Welfare Plan	Teamsters Local 237, Suffolk Regional Off-Track Betting Corporation Health and Welfare

Exemptions point to the hard fact that ACA is *not* "good for everyone." Those who voted the law in and granted these exemptions knew it—even then.

Obamacare, Obama-Insurance, "ObamaTax"

At a campaign stop on October 4, 2008, then-Senator (D-IL) Barack Obama told supporters that, "Health care should never be purchased with tax increases on middle-class families." He was being disingenuous. His namesake law is, more than anything else, a tax increase on the middle-class.

If you read the ACA (I do not recommend it), you will see that it is, more than anything else, a tax bill. It imposes several large tax increases on the middle-class. After all, as Washington privately admits, "that is where the real money is."

The following list shows the twelve new taxes created by ACA, and the four existing taxes that are increased.[12] While many of these taxes are selective, meaning not every American will be levied with the tax, we will all feel the effects in our pocket books. The revenue generated is used to expand the bureaucracy, not to improve our health.

New taxes created by ACA	
1.	Cadillac tax
2.	Earned Income Tax
3.	Employer Mandate Tax
4.	Excise Tax on Charitable Hospitals
5.	Health Insurers Tax
6.	Innovator Drug Tax
7.	Medical Device Tax
8.	Medicare Advantage Plan Surcharge (tax)
9.	Medicine Cabinet Tax
10.	New sales tax on all health insurance plans
11.	Personal Penalty Tax, formerly the Individual Mandate
12.	Tanning Salon Tax
Existing taxes increased by ACA	
13.	"Black Liquor" (bio-fuel) Tax
14.	Blue Cross/Blue Shield Tax
15.	Medicare Payroll Tax
16.	Net Investment Income Tax
17.	HSA (Health Savings Account) Withdrawal Tax
Taxes reduced or eliminated by ACA	
	NONE

The insidious element of these taxes is what really gets me. They are "stealth" taxes. You don't think you are paying for Obamacare when your paycheck goes down or your hours are cut because of the Employer Mandate. You would never think that by choosing a charitable hospital, your cost goes up (!) because that hospital is being taxed to pay for the ACA.

You think you are being ecologically friendly by choosing bio-fuel but you are really contributing your money without knowing it to the ACA bureaucracy through the "Black Liquor" Tax.

Economists estimate that a family of four could be charged as much as $20,000 per year when ACA is fully implemented.[13] Is that what you call "affordable?"

"Relax," intones Washington in a soothing voice. "Our ACA will subsidize your insurance so the premiums will be easy to pay, and all Americans can get the care they deserve. You just have to trust me!"

ACA makes subsidies available to families of four earning up to $94,000/year. Thus, between Medicaid "free" insurance and ACA subsidies, over 70 percent of the U.S. population could receive government-subsidized health insurance.

Are you happy to be part of the thirty percent who are paying for all of that? You know what "government-subsidized" means. It means you pay.

Sylvia Maltzman is a part-time tutor at a community college in Florida. Because of her ACA subsidy, she pays $23 a month for health insurance that actually costs $498.[14] Ms. Maltzman, who has high blood pressure and arthritis, said that if the Supreme Court eliminates subsidies, she could not possibly pay for her health insurance, not on her salary.

Suppose you work as a waitress and earn $21,230 per year, placing you above the poverty line (POV) of $15,800. If you live in Alabama or any one of the other twenty-three states that did not expand their Medicaid programs, your least expensive health insurance will cost well over $200 per month, which represents more than eleven percent of your total income … just on health insurance! Hardly what anyone would consider "affordable." But subsidies should take care of it, right?

Not so fast.

Keep in mind that the *cost of insurance* has gone up tremendously.[15] Those who are Medicaid-eligible and those with subsidies may not "feel" it now. The thirty percent who pay directly feel the immediate effects of ACA, in the pocket nerve, and it hurts.[16]

Those with *free* (Medicaid) or subsidized insurance may not feel it today but they too will hurt by the end of the year seeing how empty their wallets are. After all, everyone pays those hidden taxes listed above: at the fuel pump, at the grocery store, at the charity hospital, even when you want to use your own money in your HSA to pay for care.

What do we get for these tax increases? Two things.

1. We get new insurance. The president's "better" insurance contains insurance benefits and add-ons that many of us want or need, like maternity benefits for my sixty-eight year old wife. (I wish! She doesn't!) More important, the cheapest ACA insurance (Bronze level) covers only 60 percent of your medical costs, meaning you owe forty percent of your hospital bill. This is hardly what you or I would call adequate protection against financial disaster. Isn't that what insurance is supposed to do: protect us from medical bankruptcy?

2. That additional spending on insurance goes to a bureaucracy that serves the cancer, not to providers who serve us.

Cadillac Tax

Do you drive a high-priced automobile like a Cadillac Escalade, base price: $84,000? If not, you probably think you are safe from the so-called "Cadillac Tax." Surprise! (Not a happy one.) Even if you drive a ten-year old Ford, the Cadillac Tax comes down like a hammer on you! It is amazing much deception can be found in the names that Washington uses. The so-called Cadillac Tax is a great example.

This tax was supposed to make Wall Street fat cats in their Escalades "pay their fair share"—President Obama's words, not mine.[17]

The Cadillac name refers to the quality of your insurance benefits, not the car you can afford. The people who need robust insurance benefits are those whose jobs put them at risk or whose unions negotiated very expansive (and expensive) insurance benefits packages. People like steelworkers and police patrolmen. People like autoworkers and schoolteachers. This disingenuously labeled tax hits the hard-working middle-class, not hedge fund managers or Wall Street bankers in their Escalades.

Are you a police patrolman in Massachusetts? You probably drive an American car but certainly not an Escalade, not on your salary. The Cadillac Tax will take an additional $5391 out of your paycheck.[18]

The most underpaid and simultaneously most important individuals to the future of our nation are elementary and middle school teachers. Are you one, scraping by on a salary only slightly above the poverty line? You cannot afford a Ford Focus much less an Escalade. Surely *you* won't get hit by the Cadillac Tax! Sorry, the ACA hits you smack dab in your wallet, taking out an additional $2081 per year.

Small Business

You have to wonder if the ACA has a particular bone to pick with American small business—the backbone of our economy. First, the Cadillac Tax adds a cost of $8690 *per employee* per year to them.

Next, if they fail to offer employer-supported ACA-compliant insurance to their workers, the employer is fined the paltry sum of $100/day: $36,500 per year.[19] To make matters impossible for the small business owner, if the business pays for insurance that is not ACA-compliant, the employer is fined the same $36,500 per year.[20] How is the owner of any small business supposed to keep his doors open under these conditions?!

There is only one answer: cut costs elsewhere. The only thing he can do to stay in business is to reduce labor costs. So, as a result of ACA, your salary goes down, or your hours are cut, or you lose your job entirely. It's either that or all the employees lose their jobs as the employer goes out of business.

The ACA takes billions from hardworking, middle-class Americans in order for Washington to expand the size and extend the reach of a cancerous bureaucracy.

Additional ACA Taxes

There are a number of additional ways that ACA is taking money out of your wallet without your knowing it. In addition to the Tanning Salons, the following are taxes on business that they must pass on to you the customer: Excise Tax on Charitable Hospitals, Health Insurers Tax, Medicare Advantage Surcharge, and Medicine Cabinet Tax. The administration expects to generate tens of billions out of your wallet, without your knowing it.

The Medical Device Tax is particularly problematic. It is a 2.3 percent excise tax on gross revenue. If you are a start-up company, this tax will take away the capital you need to get started. If you are established, this tax will suppress the economic urge to engage in Research and Development. Either way, We The Patients lose because there will be fewer medical miracles for us when we need them.

The House of Representatives passed a resolution to repeal the Medical Device Tax in June 2015.[21] The Senate has refused to consider it and President Obama has vowed to veto the repeal if it ever got through Congress. The Democrats never heard of a tax they did not love.

The President timed his bite out of your wallet brilliantly. The penalties start out small and manageable. The real fun begins after he leaves office in 2017. At that time, the penalty you pay for failure to purchase (very expensive) ACA insurance is $695 or 2.5 percent of your income, *whichever is greater*, up to a maximum of $2,085 per year.

Through a number of overt as well as devious maneuvers, Washington is taking boatloads of money out of our wallets. What was unaffordable before ACA is now even more unaffordable.

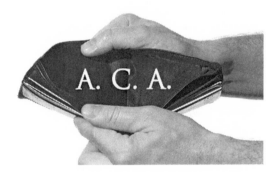

In 2014 after she felt the impact of Obamacare on her family, a private citizen named Karri Kinder posted an "Open Letter To The Obama Administration And American Citizens" that went viral.[22] Mrs. Kinder expressed a sentiment widely held in this country but not frequently extolled by the media.

After explaining how Obamacare had made her insurance situation impossible, forcing her to be dependent on government subsidies, she wrote the following.

"We just didn't want to have to be reliant on the government as we didn't have to before the ACA was passed and enacted. Seems we should have a healthcare system that maintains affordability on all levels without needing the government's funds to afford a modest lifestyle as middle-class Americans."

Mrs. Kinder concluded by confirming the evidence. "There are so many stories in my email inbox of families, just like us, getting lost in the ACA system and who were paying for their own healthcare plans that were affordable for their families until now," (following implementation of Obamacare.)

If you are not yet foaming-at-the-mouth mad, just wait.

All The Care We Deserve

President Obama repeatedly assured us that his healthcare reform would provide "all the care that Americans deserve." Apparently, we don't deserve much.

ACA cuts over $700 billion from Medicare reimbursements—money needed for care service—so it can pay for more bureaucracy: six whole new federal agencies with layers upon layers of organizational charts; implementation of 10,515 pages in the Federal Register of new rules and regulations; over a billion dollars just for a website (healthcare.gov); etc.

These actions by Obamacare proves once again this painful truth:

ACA's bureaucracy is a cancer: it takes our money and cuts our care.

From Oak Lawn, Illinois, Pastor Dan Marler shared the saga that his daughter Rachel endured because of the Affordable (No) Care Act.[23] Rachel has a genetic disorder called Smith-Magenis Syndrome that causes seizures and mental disorders along with other health problems.

When covered by pre-ACA Medicaid, Rachel was getting good care from her neurology specialist. Then the ACA came along. The doctor informed the family that he could no longer afford to see patients covered under ACA reimbursement schedules. If he did so, he couldn't pay his fixed expenses and would have to close his doors.

It gets worse. When Rachel's mother called the general physician listed on Rachel's new ACA insurance card, that doctor's office told her they too could no longer afford to accept ACA-covered patients. Note that *that* was the doctor listed on her insurance card!

And it gets even worse. When the family contacted the insurance carrier, Aetna, they were told there was no other neurologist on the panel except the one whom they had been seeing. He was still listed on their panel of specialists, even though he was not accepting ACA insured patients. What good is insurance if it doesn't get you medical care?

CoveredCalifornia is the name of the state-based Health Insurance Exchange created under ACA. When the CEO proudly announced they had signed up 2.2 million previously uninsured Californians, he failed to mention that 70 percent of the licensed physicians in the Golden State said they could not afford to see patients covered by ACA insurance, just like the doctor in Illinois caring for Rachel, the Pastor's daughter.[24]

Then there is the story of Robin Beaton who was diagnosed with an aggressive form of breast cancer.[25] She needed surgical removal of both breasts immediately, which her insurance carrier initially approved. But then, just before she went into hospital, insurance cancelled the authorization. Why? First because a report from a dermatologist whom she saw for acne three years earlier wrote that one of her spots might be precancerous. Aha!, said insurance, "Robin, you have a pre-existing condition." But, responded Robin, "ACA makes it illegal for you to deny coverage because of a pre-existing condition, which by the way, I DIDN'T have!"

Just like Rachel, the Pastor's child, Robin's story gets worse. The insurance carrier was forced to agree with Robin's comeback but still cancelled her coverage. What excuse did they use to avoid paying for very expensive surgery? They said that on a prior insurance application form Robin lied about her weight and failed to list one medication she was on. So … no surgery.

Is this the kind of care that Americans "deserve?"[26] Why, you plead with Washington, are you cutting my care? Their answer resides in three seemingly innocuous words: Cost cutting measures.

We all remember then-Speaker of the House Nancy Pelosi on the Charlie Rose TV show. She promised that ACA would "cut costs and save us all money!" There was of course President Obama's assurance that his cost cutting reforms would put $2500 back into the wallets of all Americans.

How does Obamacare intend to cut costs? First, Washington *never* cuts costs; it reduces spending, which is most definitely not the same thing. Government reduces spending on service through diversion, taking from one area to spend in another. In healthcare, Washington takes from care to spend on bureaucracy. ACA gets that money in two ways—direct and indirect.

The direct way is by cutting payments to doctors through the Medicare Fee Schedule, to the tune of $716 billion. Even the laconic now-deceased Senator Everett Dirksen would consider this "real money."[27] Cutting costs this way immediately reduces patient care services dramatically. As Robert Moffit of Heritage Foundation warned Congress in 2009, "You can't get more of something [care services for patients] by paying less for it." Congress obviously ignored Mr. Moffit.

Patients are feeling the impact of ACA's cost cutting. Just ask any Medicare or Medicaid patient how easy it is to find a doctor willing and able to accept the government fee schedules. Or just watch the flood of doctors moving out of clinical practice. American patients are beginning to experience the intolerable wait times that both Canadian citizens and our own veterans have endured for years, dying while waiting in line, so-called death by queueing.

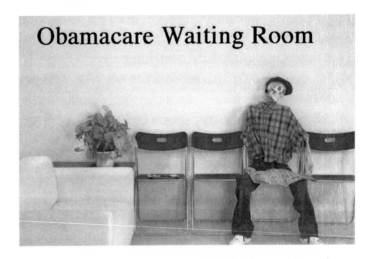

Obamacare Waiting Room

ACA has a second, indirect and well-hidden way to cut costs: IPAB. Shrouded in secrecy and immune to oversight, IPAB members—mostly lawyers, bureaucrats, administrative physicians, and doctors of alternative medicine—will decide your fate. They will say which expensive treatments are Cost Effective and which are not. The latter will not be authorized and therefore you cannot get them.

If you are either a patient or a doctor, pay close attention.

Patient: IPAB's decisions are based on effect on the budget, not medical effect on you. Something like kidney dialysis might be medically effective in saving your life but would be denied to you when it is declared Not Cost Effective. As a result, you die when you could have been saved. Is this "all the care Americans deserve?!"

Doctor: A government agency, the IPAB, is now telling you what you can do and more importantly, what you cannot do.[28] Who is practicing medicine on your patient?

As of this writing, I have been unable to discover what decisions IPAB has made. That is troubling both as a patient and a physician. Absent the facts, we must fall back on reason and past history.

I am very much afraid that IPAB will create a holocaust of the *expensives*, a class of patients I warned in a 2013 article about IPAB.[29] In the 1940's Nazi Death camps killed millions whom they called "undesirables," viz., Jews, Gypsies, and other non-Aryans. The 21st century undesirables (per IPAB) will be those who need costly therapies like heart surgery, dialysis, chemotherapy, and transplants.

Lest you think I exaggerate, read again about the Liverpool Care Protocol in chapter 8. Check out what the British National Health Service is currently doing and remember that the NHS was the model for Obamacare.

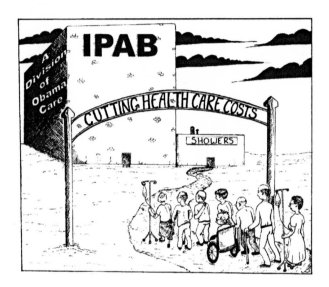

You begin to see why my blood pressure keeps rising when someone tells me how great Obamacare is. The one thing that the Affordable *Care* Act does not do is "care." The evidence proves it.

If You Like Your Doctor/Insurance, You Can Keep Them

Gloria Cantor of Florida liked her insurance and loved her doctors. After all, they were keeping her alive. Despite the President's promises, she could keep neither. In fact it was because of Obamacare that she lost both.

Gloria has cancer with tumors in both brain and bones. Mrs. Cantor and her husband, Jay, told WFTV in Orlando that they "received [a] letter in the mail [that] explains Gloria's health insurance will end next summer due to the Affordable Care Act. But after promises by President Obama … the Cantors now feel betrayed." After the insurance company dropped their old plan, it offered them a different plan that was more expensive, and would not allow Cantor to continue her care at the MD Anderson Cancer Center where Gloria has been receiving treatment for years.

Fox News host Megyn Kelly aired a different, heart-rending story of a South Carolina man, Bill Elliot, with cancer who is being forced to make what he sees as a life or death decision after his health insurance plan was cancelled because of Obamacare.[30]

Mr. Elliot, who voted for President Obama, contacted "The Kelly File" via Facebook and said he can no longer afford to pay his medical bills and does not want to take on the new costs because he does not want to put a "burden" on his family, according to *Fox News*.

Saying he feels "misled," Elliott told Kelly he liked and could afford his old insurance but, in contrast to the President's promise, he couldn't keep his insurance. His new, ACA-compliant insurance will cost him $1,500 per month with a $13,000 deductible. Elliot said he would have to opt out and pay the minimal fine for not having health insurance. Then, he "will just let nature take its course."

Have you ever asked yourself why ACA health insurance is so damned complex and confusing? You know from chapter 6 that complexity is one of bureaucracy's most powerful tools. As insurance becomes more complex, the bureaucracy wins. Why? Because then the public "needs" more rules, regulations, advisories, guidelines, explanations, and of course, more bureaucrats.

Peggy is a highly successful lawyer who needed a medical procedure. Her expensive insurance plan denied authorization and sent her an explanatory note. She read it carefully but had no idea what they were talking about.

This particular attorney went to college with the CEO of the same carrier from whom she had purchased insurance. They had remained social friends. When she called the CEO and explained the situation, he said he would gladly explain it to her. "Just FAX it over and I will call you right back." She faxed it and waited, and waited, and kept waiting.

One hour. Two hours. Three hours. Almost four hours later, he called her back.

The CEO apologized for the delay and said the following. "I read the denial and I too did not understand it. So, I called in the Director of Benefits, who had signed the letter and he could not make it understandable to me. So, I called an emergency meeting of all the Directors of our company and showed them the letter that *we* sent. When I asked what the hell it meant, there was silence. Eventually, the Head of Regulatory Compliance made things clear. He said, "They were simply following the rules and regulations set forth in the ACA. While they made no sense to anyone, our company was required to send that letter. So we did."

Think of how many bureaucrat hours were consumed—that you and I paid for—over this one issue. Now multiply that by a few trillion. That is how complexity helps the bureaucracy expand.

People often ask me why the controversy over Obamacare never seems to go away? Why does the ACA *pot* keep boiling over?[31]

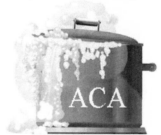

Why does it keep...?

There are the obvious reasons: Harm to the economy; pain in your wallet; loss of care; and the rise in national spending. But there is something else.

ACA is the most divisive, non-consensus driven piece of legislation, ever. It is the only piece of major social legislation passed entirely by one party over the strong objections of the other party. Not a single Republican voted for ACA. That is unheard-of. It is unique in our history.

Did you know that every, repeat every, poll taken of the American people since March 2010 has shown that more people oppose Obamacare than support it? Is it therefore a surprise that people keep trying to stop it, change it, or repeal it?

Americans oppose tyranny. That is how our country started. Even when people with power say that what they are doing "is for our own good," Americans do not like being controlled.

Americans are culturally programmed to resist coercion and Obamacare is coercion personified. It coerces the States to do what Washington wants. It coerces individuals to buy something they don't want for a price they can't afford. The coercion extends to doctors, driving them out of clinical care, leaving fewer professionals to care for more patients.

That is why the ACA pot keeps boiling over. That is why I am ready to do my Howard Beal imitation.

Do you know the 1976 iconic movie titled *Network*? Peter Finch played a TV anchorman named Howard Beal who immortalized twelve words. These are the same words I too am shouting—the same phrase you need to repeat. *"I'm mad as hell and I'm not going to take it anymore!"*

Before we discuss what we must do to rescue ourselves and our children from the cancer in healthcare, we need explore the next episode in the Obamacare soap opera—the latest Supreme Court decision.

King v. Burwell, and You

Just as this book went to press, the Supreme Court of the United States (SCOTUS) announced its decision in King v. Burwell. Their decision has not had time to impact you. Therefore, there is no evidence-of-effect; however, there is little doubt that this decision will affect every American as well as our entire nation.

Some background information will help you understand what just happened to you and what could happen in the future: A return to tyranny.

The Affordable Care Act says that subsidies to defray the increased cost of ACA-insurance coverage will be available to individuals enrolled in an Exchange "established by the State" (Sec. 1401\36B IRC, page 114). The authors of ACA expected every state to establish an exchange. After all, Washington was handing out buckets of "free" money through state-based exchanges.

Initially, only twenty-four states agreed to create Exchanges. So Washington had to create its own, *federal* exchange, called healthcare. gov. Starting in 2014, healthcare.gov began to supply billions of dollars to 7.7 million Americans to cover their health insurance premiums. For the fortunate few, out-of-pocket costs became less than $50/month for insurance premiums that actually cost more than $500/month. The difference is paid by everyone else.

Since ACA wording said only State-established exchanges could provide subsidies, the IRS issued a ruling saying that it was okay for the federal government to do likewise.

Opponents of ACA brought suit claiming that the IRS had no right to change a law that clearly states subsidies could only flow through state-established exchanges.

The four plaintiffs who brought the suit were David King, age 64, a limousine driver; Douglas Hurst, age 63, a Vietnam veteran who formerly ran a home remodeling business; Rose Luck, age 57, of Williamsburg, Virginia; and Brenda Levy, age 63, a substitute teacher. Each person qualified for subsidies, such as Mr. Hurst's out-of-pocket cost of $62.49/month for a policy that actually cost over $400/month.[32] Nonetheless, all four claimed the federal government could not legally offer subsidies, according to the ACA law.

Lawyers defending the federal government argued that ACA language was a "drafting error" and that Congress always intended to give subsidies to everyone.

Plaintiffs' lawyers said that the law as written is the law. One type of exchange—ones created by states—could legally offer subsidies, but the other, a federal exchange, could not. As Justice Anthony Scalia queried during oral arguments, "How can the *federal* government establish a *state* exchange? That is gobbledygook." (Italics per this author)[33]

Further, said plaintiffs' lawyers, the intent was clear in the language as well as in public statements made by architects of the ACA law. Limiting subsidies exclusively through state-based exchanges would provide a powerful incentive for the states to create their own exchanges.

Frankly, King v. Burwell reads like a script for a TV police drama, with accusations and charges, claims and counter-claims. Don't be surprised if, a year from now, you see a made-for-TV movie with a script based on King v. Burwell. It makes for high drama, even Greek tragedy.

After two different District Courts rendered conflicting opinions in this case, it went to the Supreme Court (SCOTUS) where oral arguments were heard on May 4, 2015. SCOTUS announced their (6-3) decision on June 25, 2015 holding for Burwell—the federal government.[34]

This decision is a victory for the Obama administration and for its progressive agenda. It is a resounding defeat for our pocket books. Much more important, it fractures the high Court's credibility and weakens our Constitution.

Over seven million Americans will continue to receive subsidies provided by Washington. Presumably, this will allow them to keep their health insurance coverage. However, the negative consequences are many.

ACA-insured patients are experiencing great difficulty finding a doctor who will accept them or the patients wait forever to get in. It will only get worse because of the federal subsidies. The problem is bureaucratic diversion (chapter 6) that keeps reducing government payments to doctors.

The American people also take a big economic "hit" as a result of the Supreme Court decision for the Obama administration. Based on a careful economic study by the American Action Forum, the following happy consequences **will not occur** because the decision for Burwell allows continuation of the financial hardships that ACA imposes on U.S. business:[35]

- 237,000 new jobs will NOT be created
- 1,270,000 workers will NOT be added to the work force
- $830-$940/year will NOT be added to every worker's paycheck
- 3,300,000 part-time workers will NOT be offered increased work hours

The 7.7 million who will continue to receive subsidies will do so at the expense of the other tax-paying Americans. There are approximately

315 million legal citizens of the United States. Only seven million receive subsidies, but every single one of us, including the seven million, will continue to pay higher and higher taxes to support those subsidies.

This is an excellent example of the President's "income redistribution" plan.

There is also a major impact of the Court's credibility, and I fear, on the integrity of the U.S. Constitution.

As the high Court judges make more and more judgments based on political leanings or personal social agendas, Americans increasingly wonder whether the high Judges remember what their "jobs" are? We expect them to do what is right, upholding the founding principles of our country enshrined in a document that starts with "We The People" through the Bill of Rights, the first ten Amendments to the Constitution.

One of Founding Fathers' key principles was the separation of powers. This was their method to prevent *concentration* of power and the inevitable tyranny that results. In an oration against aristocracy at Braintree, Massachusetts in 1772, John Adams, second President of the United States (1797-1801), said, "The only maxim of a free government ought to be to trust no man living with power to endanger the public liberty."

Separation of powers works as follows. The Legislative branch of government—Congress—makes the laws but has no power to implement them. The Executive branch—the President and all federal agencies—implement the laws as passed by Congress, but cannot change the laws or make new ones.

The Executive and Legislative branches are expected to be co-equal in authority. The power of one was supposed to balance out the power of the other. The third branch of government, the Judiciary with the Supreme Court as the pinnacle, was supposed to be the arbiter of disputes between the Executive and the Legislative branches. The Court's primary duty was to maintain the balance of power between the other two branches. The Constitution's separation of powers, a variation of Montesquieu's "checks and balances," thus weakened the potential for any one person or single group to control the people.

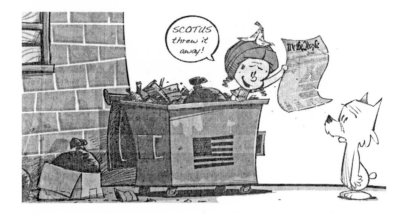

By deciding for the Obama administration, the Court encouraged the *concentration* of power within the Executive branch. It placed the White House *above* Congress rather than its equal. The Judges took a sledgehammer to the separation of powers, a pillar of American democracy. The Burwell decision pushes the U.S. president toward the status of Emperor, Caesar, Sultan, or Tzar.

In 1776, we rebelled against a tyrant named George III who had the title of King. Has the Supreme Court renamed our chief servant-of-the-people from President to Emperor? Are today's Executive Orders the modern equivalent of yesteryear's Royal Decrees?

ACA Successes & Failures

We have looked at all the evidence of what Obamacare actually did and what it was intended to do. Keep in mind that intentions of the drafters of the ACA can be (and no doubt were) both public, as in what they promised on TV and radio, and covert—as in undisclosed—outcomes they wanted but did not share with the public.

Determination of Success (S) or Failure (F) for Obamacare			
	Advertised Outcome	Actual Outcome	S	F
1	Reduce national spending	National spending increased		✓
2	Health care more affordable	Health care is less affordable		✓
3	Health care more accessible	Health care is less accessible		✓
4	Health insurance more affordable	Insurance is more expensive		✓
5	Reduce number of uninsured	More people are insured	✓	✓
6	*Not publicly discussed*	Increase government control	✓✓	
7	*Not publicly discussed*	Expand bureaucracy	✓✓	

When you compare advertised outcomes with actual ones, the failures predominate. National spending is way up: failure. Healthcare is both less available and less affordable: failure times two. Health insurance is considerably more expensive: failure.

In the summary table above, you will note that one item is both a success and a failure. The number of insured Americans has clearly increased, so that should rate a check (✓) in the success column. But most newly insured patients have great difficulty finding a doctor, and the purpose of having insurance is to get care. So if there are more insured people who *can't get care* that also requires a check on the failure side.

Obamacare has two "successes," if you want to call them that. They weren't advertised or even mentioned publicly.

First, in the most highly regulated industry in the country, namely healthcare, Obamacare has had great success in extending government control. Washington tells sellers of insurance what they must sell. The federal government tells sellers of services, doctors and nurses, what they will be paid. Washington also tells consumers what they must purchase, or else. ACA's IPAB tells doctors what they can and cannot do for patients. This is effectively total control of healthcare and deserves two checks in the success column.

The second "success," also worthy of two check marks, is ACA's massive expansion of the bureaucracy. Along with greater control, that is precisely what the cancer wants.

Final Scorecard For Obamacare

Even as American medicine was creating miracles in health care *service*, the healthcare *system* was sickening, weakening, and failing. This has been going on for decades.

Doctor Obama said he had the cure and called it Obamacare. The *doctor* assured us that his therapy would heal patient Healthcare. We just had to trust him. His treatment has now been started. We can see what it has done to the patient.

Based on the evidence, we must conclude that Obamacare is poison, not panacea.[36] ACA is cancer of greed and power at its worst: it takes our money and cuts our care.

What About Us?

It is more exciting and certainly easier to score the *game* called healthcare than to keep track of the *successes* and *failures* of our healthcare system. We know every two years whether Republicans or Democrats are ahead. We can easily see whether the pharmaceutical company wins or the medical malpractice lawyer.

We must resist keeping score on a daily basis and focus on the big, long-term picture. What about us? Are we winning or losing?

The system we call healthcare is supposed to keep We The Patients healthy or restore our health when we are ill. That is what "winning" looks like. Unfortunately, the American healthcare system itself is sick. It has cancer. As the cancer grows, the system can no longer do what it is supposed to do: care for us. As the cancer grows, We The Patients lose. We die.

When we look back at what Washington has done over the years to treat our sick healthcare system, we can see that they have all failed. Regardless of whether the approach was economic, political, ethical or historical, healthcare has gotten worse and the cancer has grown. The latest "reform" bill, Obamacare, is hastening healthcare's march to the gallows and taking us with it.

Two things need to change: how we think, and how the healthcare system works. In chapter 10, we will learn to *think* for ourselves. In chapter 11, we will discover what we can *do* to create a simple healthcare system, one that works for us and not for the cancer.

TEN

First Steps

A while ago, a story circulated around the Internet. Conservatives loved it—said it captured the essence of the problem of Obamacare. Liberals despised it saying that it is immoral to question everyone's right to health care.

Here's a version of what was circulated. The author is anonymous, so I felt free to alter the story a bit. The events in this story didn't happen; rather it's an allegory, a representation of an idea through a group of characters:[1]

> A group of diverse young people had taken over a large corner section of our local Starbucks. While drinking more caffeine than was good for them, my friend Paul overheard one exclaim, "Isn't Obama like God or Jesus Christ? I mean, after all, like Jesus, he is out there healing the sick with free care, throwing out the money lenders, and getting us what we are all entitled to!"
>
> A young woman loudly agreed, "Yeah, and *He* is doing this for nothing. I cannot believe anyone would think that the free market works in health care."
>
> A third chimed in, "The greedy Republicans don't want to pay for the health care we are entitled to. They just want to make more money. Obama should be made a saint after

what he did for us, especially for the less fortunate." At that point, Paul could remain silent no longer.

Mustering all the restraint Paul could find, he stood up, walked over to their table, and spoke up. "Excuse me, may I join you?" They smiled and welcomed him to their conversation. After marshaling his thoughts, he began to speak to the entire group.

"I couldn't help overhear your conversation. I am going to give one of you my brand new car parked out front. Nice, isn't it? Less than a thousand miles on it! It will cost you nothing. I will pay all of the expenses, including gas. Anyone interested?" They looked at each other and then at him in astonishment.

Paul repeated himself. "I am quite serious. I will give you my car for free, no money whatsoever. Anyone interested?" In unison, they all shouted, "Hell, Yeah!"

Paul went on. "Since there are many of you and there is only one car, I will have to choose one person. I will give it to whomever is most willing to obey the rules of the contract." They looked at one another, an expression of bewilderment on their faces.

A perky young woman asked, "What are the rules?"

Paul smiled and said, "I don't know yet. I have not decided. Let's sign the contract and then I will figure out what the terms and rules will be later. However, a free car is a free car."

They giggled amongst themselves. The youngest said, "What a crazy old coot. Go take your meds, old man."

Paul took out his keys, leaned over their table, and went on. "I am serious, this is a legitimate offer." They gaped at him for a moment.

"I'll take it, you old fool. Give me the keys," exclaimed the most brazen of the young men.

"Then I presume you accept my terms?" Paul asked.

"Oh hell yeah! Sure, absolutely! Where do I sign?"

Paul took a pen, grabbed a brown napkin, and wrote, "I give to (___fill in your name___) my car for free. He has no financial obligation whatsoever, so long as he accepts and abides by all the terms and rules that I will set forth later." Paul signed it, told the young man to write in his name, and sign it, which he did.

"Are these the keys to my fancy new vehicle?" he asked in a mocking tone of voice. All eyes were on Paul as he pushed back from the table, arose, and dangled them before the new owner.

"Now that you have signed the contract, I will tell you the rules and regulations you must obey. You are entitled to drive it only one day a week and never on weekends. You may not eat or drink anything inside the car. Oh, and you will obey me without question, no matter what I say or do. You will vote as I tell you and think as I tell you. Those are the terms you have accepted. Here are your keys."

He looked at me dumbfounded. "Are you out of your mind? Who would ever agree to those ridiculous terms?" the young man shouted.

"You just did," Paul calmly said, "when you thought you could get something for 'free,' you gave up your freedom to choose by signing a contract where the terms had not been clearly specified on advance. By accepting a free car with an open-ended contract, you committed yourself to do anything I say."

"You can shove that stupid deal up your a** old man, I want no part of it," exclaimed the now infuriated young man.

"Wait just a minute!! You have committed yourself to this deal. Your friends all witnessed it. Maybe I won't let you out of it. You chose blindly and without thought, to give up your ability to choose, your freedom, in exchange for a free car. You must now do whatever I tell you. I am your master. You are my slave. You can call me, oh, let me think, I like the title of ... President."

After a few moments of yelling, unrepeatable comments, and various slurs, Paul revealed his true purpose: "What I did to you is what Congress, the President (whom you said is a saint,) and their henchmen bureaucrats did to all of us. They suckered us with their so-called 'Affordable Health Care Act.' Only after they signed away our freedom to choose did we start seeing what it would really do to us. Only after they got our hopes up did we learn that we weren't the winners. Not until they started actually building this thing did we find out that far too much of the money we've paid supposedly for health care actually goes to the bureaucracy. They have taken our money yet we do not get the care we need, *that we paid for.* ACA is spending money we don't have, and so we are passing on a huge bill for our children to pay.

"We mistakenly thought that we could get something for nothing. We bought in to the fantasy that there really is a 'free lunch.' We got suckered into accepting an entitlement that we did not earn. Worst of all, we traded our most precious possession, freedom, for a mirage generated by a greedy, power hungry, out-of-control bureaucracy."

Paul tore up the napkin contract, kept his car keys, and walked out hoping that he had helped the young people begin to think for themselves.

It doesn't matter if you are a conservative, or liberal, or socialist, or libertarian, or independent, or, or, or, we *all* need health care eventually. We *all* feel BARRC's bite—the mind-numbing forms, the endless red tape, the constant demand for more money (read "taxes") to pay for more and more bureaucracy.

We Americans are in a tough spot. Our healthcare system hasn't provided us the care we need for many years. Now we are paying insurance premiums far higher than we had been, and somehow seven million of the poorest Americans think they will get health care while those of us who pay and pay can't find a doctor.

Because we didn't like what we had before ACA, like the kids in the free car story, we bought the lie—and it wasn't that healthcare was going to be "free" (even though that was the buzz on the street up until the bill was in its final stages of being pushed through Congress). We were told that because our insurance premiums were too high and that there were poor people who couldn't get decent care, the lie we heard was that healthcare "reform" was going to be *great*. Some questioned, others didn't. Some demanded proof. Others said "Proof, schmoof, who needs it? If the president says it's great, it must be great. He understands me and cares about me, so I trust him."

In the end, just like the young man in the free car story, we allowed our lawmakers to sign a blank check made out to the "cancer of bureaucratic greed." And only now are we finding out what they *bought* in our name: more bureaucrats and fewer doctors. Only now are we beginning to experience what the cancer, through its ACA, is doing to us and to our great nation.

In this book, I intentionally tried to keep political name-calling and blaming to a minimum. When I complain how bad Obamacare is for us that is because I am a doctor. My focus is strictly *medical*, not political. I am neither a Republican nor a Democrat. I support whatever works to make a patient better. I oppose what doesn't. If Obamacare were good for the health of We The Patients, I would be all for it. The ACA is poison and that is why I am against it. I am simply trying to do the best I can for the patient known as Healthcare.

If healthcare is critically ill (it is), and Obamacare isn't the cure (it isn't) then what should we do? The first step is to find ways to think for ourselves by looking past all the hype, propaganda, infomercials, and outright lies. The second step is to take back control. We will discuss the former here and now. Taking back control is the subject of the last chapter.

Think For Yourself: Truth or Disinformation?

What is truth and what are the lies surrounding healthcare? As you answer this vital question, you need to be aware of something. There are powerful forces on both sides of the political spectrum that "spin" the information that you're getting. Spin is simply how something is presented to you, like virtually any commercial on T.V. Spin becomes sinister when it takes on the form of disinformation.

Disinformation is false data. It' not just a lie. It is not even a "big lie," the kind of lie that makes you gasp at its audacity and question your own sanity because it's so outrageous. Rather, disinformation is a *series of lies* that are made to look deceptively like truth. These lies are spread deliberately in a carefully planned program, repeated loudly and frequently, over and over from media point to media point, indeed on as many communication channels as the bureaucracy controls. Disinformation is put forth as truth, talked about as truth, spreads as though it were incontestable truth, yet it doesn't make sense. It doesn't add up and when you try to apply it or put it into effect you fail, in some circumstances, catastrophically.

Disinformation is a pattern of lies that is spread deliberately for some hidden purpose. In the case of poor healthcare, disinformation is one of the main tools used by the cancer of greed, right alongside intentional complexity.

Disinformation is "bigger" than the biggest of single lies. And even though it doesn't make sense to you, after a while, because you hear it so much, you begin to question your own judgment. You substitute someone else's choices for your own, and that is what makes disinformation so dangerous.

In the book *1984*, the people were constantly bombarded with slogans like "Freedom is slavery" and "Ignorance is strength." While this made no sense to them, eventually they began to accept the slogans on faith. After all, Big Brother kept saying it and everyone believed Big Brother cared for them. So they disregarded their own judgment and common sense and accepted disinformation as truth. They trusted the disinformation instead of trusting themselves.

When President Obama said that U.S. healthcare costs must be cut and that spending was on an "unsustainable" trajectory, he spoke a *truth*. This made sense, and you could easily prove it for yourself.

When President Obama assured us that ACA would make health insurance affordable, then later said that we "could keep our doctor if we liked him" and even later declared that his reform would reduce healthcare spending, he was spreading a Big Lie. Though our own minds told us that more spending wouldn't *reduce* spending, because he sounded so convincing and caring, many accepted what he said "on faith."

When the President said in 2008 during his first election campaign: "When you spread the wealth around, it's good for everybody," that was classic disinformation.[2] It sounded too good to be true (and is). Your mind screamed at you: "TANSTAAFL (there ain't no such thing as a free lunch"). However, between the constant drumbeat, the demand for orthodoxy (never question the person with the big title and sonorous voice), and with everyone seeming to whisper in your ear, "who are you to argue with the President and all those politicos standing in front of a bank of microphones," what were you supposed to believe?

Worse, disinformation squashes you if you try to speak out. Try saying something like "Wait a minute. That doesn't add up. That doesn't make sense." You are instantly lambasted for not being a "solid citizen" and for not "being with the program." You are made to feel guilty for "refusing to do your part" to take care of the less fortunate.

Here's another oft-cited bit of disinformation: "If you're against Obamacare you're against Obama and if you are against Obama, you must be a racist." That one always makes me shudder. It effectively shuts down any kind of dialogue because no one wants to be labeled a racist. And that is the precise goal of disinformation—to shut down opposition, to silence the voice of dissent, to kill any plan other than preserving the "status quo" and helping the cancer.

Disinformation is an insidious tool used liberally by both political parties in service of the cancer. If we're going to do anything about it, we have to recover our ability to look and think for ourselves. That requires education to recognize the disinformation. But we also need to combat it. That requires guts.

Think For Yourself: Resist Groupthink

There is another force at work here, one that is related to disinformation. As you decide about ACA, you need to be mindful of groupthink.

Groupthink is when the "mob mentality" takes over rational thinking. You think a certain way because others think that way, even though if you stepped far enough back from the group and looked at what you were thinking and saying (like if you oppose Obama then you are automatically a racist) you would see how odd it all is.

Groupthink is a way that members of a group minimize disagreement, discord, and the anxiety produced by conflict and controversy. The easy way to have a friendly committee meeting is to agree with those who speak the loudest or who sit at the head of the table. Groupthink is uniformity of thought within a group. It is political correctness and conformity made manifest. On Maslow's famous Hierarchy (Pyramid) of Needs, groupthink satisfies our need to feel safe and to belong.[3]

If the goal of a gathering is to minimize stress, then groupthink is the right approach. However, if the purpose is to make the best decision, then the last thing you want is groupthink. By suppressing views that differ with accepted wisdom, groupthink limits the options for problem solving.

When there is groupthink, the "logical," "obvious," indeed *only* answer is the answer that goes along with all the other answers that have been given for however long, meaning that it just goes along with the status quo, even if the status quo isn't working. In other words, groupthink is really our being lazy and taking a stance of I'll-just-go-along-with-everyone-else-in-order-to-get-along. Taken to the extreme, however, it can result in lynching and riots.

Envision a Congressional budget committee or better yet, an IPAB meeting where the problem is too many requested services for the resources allocated. The groupthink answers are (a) cut the services; (b) spend more money, or (c) both. No one would dare suggest there might be some way to (d) increase services without spending more; (e) to cut spending while maintaining current service level; or best of all, (f) both increase services while simultaneously reducing costs.

Groupthink would never allow someone to suggest the possibility of d, e, or f. That is why Joel Brenner's work (the doctor in Camden, New Jersey), showing that better and cheaper are simultaneously possible in healthcare, has received so little media attention. It is counter to groupthink. It exposes the disinformation.

Groupthink promotes disinformation. To avoid being deceived, we need to be constantly vigilant, recognize disinformation when it is offered, reject it, and make decisions based solely on our own thought processes and conclusions.

Think For Yourself: You Are A "Thinking System"

When you look in the mirror, you see a human being, not a system. But in fact *you are a system*. A system is defined as a set of connected parts that interact with each other, and those interactions produce the system's outcomes. There are mechanical systems like a car or a chemical reaction. Unless it is broken or wears out, a mechanical system will produce the same outcome every time (like when you add one hydrogen atom to two carbon atoms, you get H_2O every time without fail.)

Then there is something called a complex adaptive systems. These systems are only biological in nature, like an ant or an elephant, and as the name says, they adapt. An ant can learn, for example, but only by trial and error. It doesn't plan how or what it will learn. Ants do have free will: they choose where to go and what to eat. Ants can leave trails of smell information and thus teach other ants where to find food. In this way, ants can adapt to the local environment.

Your body is a complex adaptive system. Your kidneys, liver, brain, heart and muscles are some of the parts. The kidneys cleanse the blood that the heart circulates. The blood contains the energy needed by the muscles, energy that the liver made. The brain tells your legs where (and how) you should walk.

We are not just our bodies, however. We are unique. Experts in system dynamics call us "thinking systems" but maybe better phrases would be mindful systems, or systems-with-souls.[4] We have all the capabilities of a complex adaptive system, but humans have two additional, unique features, which flowers, ants, and elephants do not. These unique attributes give us the ability to be great and to be terrible, even at the same time.

First, thinking systems can "program" themselves. Neither a mountain lion, nor a computer (even with Apple's operating system of the same name) can do that. We can plan how to learn and decide in advance what we will learn. Complex adaptive systems have only trial and error; we have structured learning. Migratory birds, for example, took perhaps millions of years to learn to fly in a "V" formation because those who did survived the most and were able to procreate. Tour de France bicycle racers figured out the same aerodynamics the first time they raced.

Bicycling teams plan ways to study (and learn) how to make their riding most efficient. They do tests in wind tunnels and on the road. They develop ways to get their team leader to the finish line first. Sometimes, their need to win gets the better of another need—to be honest. I need only mention Lance Armstrong who won the Tour de France seven consecutive years (1999-2005) but later had these titles stripped as he was forced to admit that he was guilty of blood doping.

Structured, purposeful learning—self-programming—gives humans (thinking systems) the ability to cure cancer, to love, to invent amazing things. It also allows us to make better, more efficient ways to lie, cheat, poison ourselves, or kill someone else.

The second feature unique to thinking systems is goal setting. We humans can create multiple goals for ourselves. All other complex adaptive systems have one goal and one goal only: survival. While that is our goal as well, we also are compelled to do more. We can decide to paint a great work of art or run faster than anyone else.

We can also decide that our honor and our self-determination (the right to choose our own destinies) are more important than endangering our lives. No lion would ever run in to a burning building to save some other lions he had never met. The New York City Firefighters knew the risk they were taking on 9/11 and chose to go in anyway. They had a larger goal than their own survival—saving others. A suicide bomber too has a personal goal that is more important than his life. No cow would ever strap a bomb to her belly.

Thinking systems are capable of true greatness. We are also able, sometimes simultaneously, to convince ourselves to do terrible things to ourselves and to others. No cow would ever light up a cigarette. Lions eat only what they need, never so much that they become morbidly obese. Humans do both: we smoke and gorge ourselves.

Great and/or terrible: we are thinking systems. We have goals of our own. We may accept the goals of others or we may choose to reject them. Here's the key: As long as we remain free thinking persons, we control ourselves.

When we trade away our freedom, say to the cancer of bureaucracy, we give up control. We hear the siren song of disinformation: "Lay down the burden of responsibility. I will make your dreams come true. I will give you everything you are entitled to, everything you so richly deserve. Just give up your personal power to choose and let the bureaucracy make all your choices for you." What happens? The rational part of us shuts down. We become "hypnotized," in a way and follow that call.

To restore our freedom and regain our health, we must wrest control back from the cancer. We must own up to the fact that we can and must think for ourselves, no matter what the group might say and not matter how dangerous it might seem.

What Does It Mean To Be Free?

Being free means being able to choose for yourself. Being free means you decide. You can go where you want or stay where you are. You can eat what you want, when you want. You have the right to dissent, to speak your mind, to defend yourself against someone trying to harm you, including a tyrannical government. Our Constitution guarantees a very specific number of rights, and we believe that these rights are inalienable—no one can take them away from us.

To be free means you are self-determined. You get to do what you want, have what you want, stay where you want. The key: It's your choice, and you have the right to decide who you are, what you do, and what you have. However, never for a moment buy into the idea that anyone has a right to drive a Mercedes or even a Ford. No one has a "right" to own a car, a five-bedroom house, or to have a four-week vacation in Disneyland. It is perfectly fine to want those things. It is even better to go and earn the wherewithal (literally the cash) to have and do these things—and you most certainly have the right to do that.

To be a free person means that you decide for yourself. Being free is hard. It requires strength. Being free to decide means considering evidence, exercising our right to inspect data, pushing away the comforting embrace of groupthink, and doing that continually.

When you decide for yourself, you are in control of yourself. When you fall into the trap of letting others think for you—which is the trap of disinformation and groupthink—then you're sunk. You've allowed yourself to become enslaved to someone else: Their ideas, their choices, and their decisions *for you.*

Doesn't sound very palatable, does it?

This is why it is so vital for you to learn how to recognize disinformation. Just because someone with a big title said it, doesn't make it true. Just because I authored over four hundred articles on healthcare doesn't mean you should accept what I write *without reservation.* You must always question and verify. Never take anything or anyone on faith.

We either decide *for ourselves* what is true, or we accept what others say and suffer the consequences of their choices.

Freedom Comes With Responsibility

In her 1960 book titled *You Learn by Living: Eleven Keys for a More Fulfilling Life,* Eleanor Roosevelt wrote the following. "Freedom makes a huge requirement of every human being. *With freedom comes responsibility.* [Italics are mine.] For the person who is unwilling to grow up, the person who does not want to carry his own weight, this is a frightening prospect."

When you are free, you are not only able to choose, you know you have to. Even if you decide not to choose, *that* in itself is a choice. The one who is free is the one who decides for—is in control of—himself or herself. Freedom means choosing. And when you choose, you accept the consequences of your choice. So, freedom means accepting responsibility.

Responsibility isn't blame. It's the simple admission that, "I did that." Here's how the two work together: You make the choice, "I want freedom." But as soon as you choose, those who don't want you to have freedom hit you in the face with accusations made acceptable through disinformation and group think. Instead of withdrawing from that (which may be your first tendency), as a free and responsible person, you stand up and say, "I did that, and I stand by the fact that I chose."

I'm not writing anything new. Over three hundred years ago, one of the founders of liberal thinking, Thomas Hobbes, wrote this in his allegory *The Leviathan*. For human beings to claim rights without accepting responsibility for their choices, "would be absurd, just as it would be absurd to expect carnivores might reject meat or fish stop swimming."[5]

A U.S. Founding Father warned us about the person who refuses to accept the responsibility with the famous quote, "Those who surrender freedom for security will not have, nor do they deserve either one." Historians argue who said it: Benjamin Franklin or Thomas Jefferson. However, there is no doubt that it was Jefferson who wrote, "The price of freedom is eternal vigilance."

Let me put this as bluntly and succinctly as I can: *You cannot have one—freedom—without the other—responsibility.* They are a package deal. They always come together.

What Is The Opposite Of Being Free?

What is the opposite of freedom? Slavery. In a free society, *no one* has the right to control another person against their will: That is the essence of being free. To control someone else who does not voluntarily relinquish control is to enslave him or her.

One of the big debates that persist about health care is whether or not it is a right. I touched on this in chapter 8. The right to health care seems to be an accepted part of groupthink, and some of my colleagues in medicine subscribe to it. However, when I point out to them that such a right takes away their right to choose, their very freedom, and makes them slaves of their patients, they generally become incensed and defensive. However, after they think for themselves a bit, I routinely hear, "You're right. Health care shouldn't be a right. In fact, it cannot be, not if I am to remain a free woman (or man)."

You cannot demand service at a restaurant, a store, or a lawyer's office. If the server, storeowner, or lawyer *must* give you service, then that person is no longer free. You pay for the wait staff to bring your food, for the salesperson to show you various goods, or for the lawyer to prepare a legal document. Those services are voluntary, both by you and by them.

Now let's look at health care. After all, it is a commercial service provided by one person to another. It is voluntary by both people. But if healthcare is considered a right, then a patient has a "right" to demand service from a provider and that provider does not have the right to refuse. This means the provider is no longer free.

Anyone who says you are "entitled" (meaning you have a right) to health care must then advocate a return to slavery for doctors, nurses, and therapists. There is no other logical conclusion. If you don't believe me, go and demand service from your doctor (or better your lawyer) as your right, and then refuse to pay him. See what happens.

The Trap of Population Medicine

At this moment in time, you have a choice about your healthcare—not as much as you used to, but you still have options. The two choices are these: *personal medicine*—you decide for you—or *population medicine*—a bureaucrat decides for all of us, you included.

Let me be crystal clear. Population medicine is what they have in universal care countries such as Great Britain and Canada. Population medicine is where the U.S. is headed under the ACA law. The government bureaucracy decides what care will be made available based on their national budgetary commitments. If your health problem is too expensive, or your treatment is deemed Not Cost Effective, you are denied that care, even if it would save your life. If you want proof and can stomach it, re-read the section on the Liverpool Car Protocol in chapter 8.

When people tell you that Canadians and Britons are happy with their care, ask the people in those countries who are older, have chronic conditions, are not legal citizens, or need very costly care. They are not happy with their care because they don't get it. They are victims of population medicine.

Think about your father or aunt or grandmother, with kidney failure or heart disease. Do you want to condemn them to die? I doubt it. With personal medicine, they have choices. With population medicine, neither they nor you are free to choose.

So, do you want what is best for you *decided by you*, or do you want what is "best for you" *decided by someone else*, based on what he or she thinks is best for the national budget, not for you? Do you choose personal medicine or population medicine? Unfortunately, that is a decision you can no longer make. ACA, now the law of the land, has taken your power of choice away from you. The IPAB bureaucracy, an integral part of the ACA law, decides what health care you will get (or won't). You no longer have the right to choose. You no longer are free. Is that what you want? Is that what you expected?

The Government Will Never Cure Its Own Cancer

We all want to be free. We all want to live long and prosper. But did you realize that you *need* freedom in order to "live long and prosper?" Do you realize that when your freedom is taken away, your health goes with it? That is the way cancer kills you, by taking away your freedom.

Throughout this book, I have been using the analogy that healthcare has cancer. Greed in the commercial world—insurance companies and pharmaceuticals—is usually benign, constrained by both free market forces and federal regulations. But the cancer in government is not constrained by those forces and certainly government does not regulate itself. So, the cancer in the government bureaucracy that controls healthcare is, in reality, killing the patient—both the healthcare system and We The Patients.

I have said it numerous times, but it bears repeating: Bureaucratic greed is lethal.[6] It serves only the bureaucracy and in fact, does so at the expense of the consumer and society. When ACA takes billions of dollars away from health care services to pay for more healthcare bureaucracy, that is not helping us—that is killing us.

Bureaucracy-with-power is what we call government. That bureaucracy is riddled with cancer of a most virulent, malignant form. By taking away our freedom, it takes away our health. Watch the process in action in the following illustration:

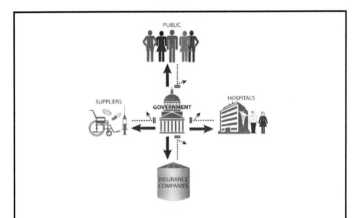

The Capitol dome in the center is, of course, the Federal government. The solid arrows (→) reflect communication and control from the government to We The Public and all the other components of the healthcare industry. The dashed arrows (------>) are our attempts to communicate with the Government, but they are blocked as shown by the (||) symbol.

As you can see by the solid arrows, the government, through BARRC and the control of the money flow, controls doctors, hospitals, insurance companies, suppliers (including providers), as well as the public—you and me. The bureaucracy (government) says what all these entities must do; how much they can charge; how much they will receive; and what health care services will (or won't) be provided.

The dashed arrows indicate attempts by doctors, hospitals, insurance, suppliers, and the public to influence government actions. The problem is, these efforts are blocked (represented by the || symbols). Through BARRC, bureaucracy has created a one-way flow of communication: orders from the government that we must accept. This is hardly what one would call "representative" government.

The solution is clear from the diagram. The blocks must be abolished. Communication must go both ways. Most important, *control* (the bigger, solid arrows) should be in our hands, not the bureaucracy's greedy paws. We need to retake our freedom, our control. It's that simple, and it's that hard.

No cancer will ever cure itself. Yet, we seem to be expecting just that! We look to the government to cure the cancer of bureaucratic greed, yet government is totally controlled by that greed. Bureaucratic greed will never cut itself out!

Do you really think that by asking nicely, a cancerous tumor or a tapeworm parasite will say, "Yeah, sure, of course, I will go away. I will give you back control of your body and the resources you need that I have been stealing. No problem!"

Not a chance.

YOU Are The Doctor

If we keep waiting for someone else, anyone else, to fix healthcare for us, we are "Waiting For Godot"—it will never happen.[7] What are we going to do? We have to do it ourselves. We have to save ourselves, from our own sick healthcare system.

We do not have the luxury of saying, "It's not my job. It's someone else's responsibility." You are a free man or woman. You take responsibility.

I hope you accept the folly of saying, "That's the government job." It's not. It's ours—yours and mine, because government bureaucracy IS the problem. The current healthcare system will never fix itself. You know that is true. Just look at what the bureaucrats have done to healthcare over the past fifty years. Why would you ever expect cancer to go away voluntarily?

You also need to have faith in your ability to think for yourself. It is deadly to say, "There must be someone more qualified than me!" Ask yourself, who is better able than you to decide your life or your death?

Accept it! YOU are the doctor for sick Healthcare. You are already way ahead of the self-styled "physicians" (the bureaucrats) who have been treating this patient so badly.

YOU think for yourself. (They don't.)

YOU know your enemy. (They are the cancer and they see you as the enemy.)

YOU choose in your own best interest. (You are most qualified.)

YOU decide instead of following the orders of the cancer.

You also understand that greed is a part of who we humans are. We are all greedy, to greater or lesser extents. No one is a saint.

You cannot cut out (eliminate) greed.

However, what if "greed" were aligned with the outcomes we want? What if those greedy doctors and venal hospitals were paid extra, not for "performance," but for our good health? What if those greedy insurance companies were rewarded with profit, i.e., with money, when we stayed healthy and lived longer? What if the greedy White House or Congress got a performance bonus—let's call it re-election—only when our national productivity and our global competitiveness increase?

There are ways to use our desire for profit and power to create win-win scenarios instead of the win-lose we have now. You first have to believe that it is possible.

Then you have to demand real data, not empty promises. You need to demand that our law makers show us evidence that what they say will happen has happened in the past and will happen in the future. Don't let them pass a law without proof-of-effect in hand.

If we had just demanded such proof before Washington passed EMTALA, HIPAA, or ACA, we wouldn't be in the pickle we are now in.

First Actions

So how do we fix healthcare? In a way, you already know the answer. We need to put people in positions of power who are going to rein in the cancer and give control back to us. To do that, however, starts with some of the simplest yet hardest actions a human being can undertake. Here they are:

Think And Discuss

Earlier in this chapter, I gave you a number of techniques to help you think for yourself, from recognizing disinformation through resisting groupthink to accepting your pre-eminent status as a thinking system. Now it is time for you to do it: Think for yourself.

John F. Kennedy said, "Without debate, without criticism, no administration and no country can succeed—and no republic can survive." To debate and critique what the government does requires that we think for ourselves.

A century before Kennedy, a great nineteenth century American thinker, Ralph Waldo Emerson, said that to achieve what we want for ourselves, we must become "Man Thinking." By that he meant someone who thinks and decides for himself or herself, rather than parroting the thoughts of others, and thus, making oneself a "victim of society" (Emerson's words again).[8]

Think about Emerson's courage and his political *in*correctness. He was giving that lecture before a group of college students on the eve of the Civil War, when our country was completely polarized. This was a time when rational discourse was impossible—about slavery, freedom, morality, or anything else for that matter. You did not dialogue with opposing positions. You shouted at them and eventually shot at them. You did not question or think for yourself. You were on one side or the other, without thought or reservation.

Into that cauldron comes Emerson saying, in essence, *throw away your books, ignore what your teachers tell you, reject what your superiors declare, and think for yourselves!*

Look, Don't Listen!

Come with me for a moment outside the U.S., specifically to Istanbul, Turkey. I was there in June 2013 during the commencement of the popular uprisings. I heard on the radio what then-Prime Minister Tayyip Erdoğan said was happening, translated word for word by my son. I also saw first-hand what the protesters were actually doing, and more importantly what they weren't doing.

What I saw did not connect with what I heard. What I heard was spun, false, and in many instances completely fabricated. This point is important.

For example, I personally *heard* the Prime Minister say that the protesters were "hooligans who urinated and defecated in public parks," and they incited the violence with the police simply responding. This was reported on radio, TV, and in all the newspapers.

However when I *looked* for myself, I saw something quite different. I watched completely peaceful and respectful people gather to "petition the government for redress of grievances." [First Amendment to the U.S. Constitution] They brought flowers to honor those who had already died. The police brought a water cannon filled with pepper spray and tear gas. (I know this directly, as I was gassed.)

Oh, I also saw the portable toilets ("Porta-Potties") that the protesters brought with them because they knew that the police had closed the public bathrooms. That is where they defecated and urinated.

The Prime Minister spoke, and I could recognize it as disinformation because I looked, I did not just listen. "Look, don't Listen" means confirm for yourself. Do not accept as true what others say is true. Everyone— even your friends but especially those in power—has their own agenda. You must figure out what is really true, free from "spin," before you can decide what to do about it: Support, oppose, or do nothing.

Thomas Jefferson said, "An informed citizenry is the only true repository of the public will." If We The People really want to be in control and if we want to be free, we cannot let others manipulate us by giving us their "altered" reality and expect us to swallow it whole.

When I used "Look, Don't Listen" in Turkey, I *heard* a lie but *saw* the truth. I could tell the difference because I looked for myself.

"Know Thy Enemy."

At a recent town hall meeting on healthcare (what else?), I had finished my formal remarks and asked the audience for their thoughts, comments, or questions. One of the attendees arose to ask quite calmly, "Do you believe that the bureaucracy is evil? Is it the Devil?" (The town hall was sponsored by a religion-based organization.)

I answered his question with a question. "In the movie *Finding Nemo*, do you blame the shark for trying to eat the adorable but forgetful fish named Dory? Of course, you don't. The shark is just behaving according to its nature. Its biologic instructions command it to eat anything it can."

The bureaucracy is like the shark. It is not inherently evil. It is just doing what its DNA tells it to do. In computer language, it is just following the programming code. However, the instructions built into bureaucracy are different from biologic organisms in one subtle but very important way. Animals are programmed to survive so they can procreate and continue their species. Bureaucracy is made up of people—some well-meaning, some just doing their jobs, and some who are driven by greed. Together they make up an entity called the bureaucracy, which has developed cancer. That cancer has reprogrammed the entire bureaucracy to grow and expand. Those who run the bureaucracy buy into the myth that survival requires continuous expansion.

Earlier in this chapter, we learned that humans are unique. We are thinking systems and therefore different from all other animals. We are the only self-programming beings on the planet. You tell yourself what to do. You need not respond to internal instructions, like a shark, a computer, or the bureaucracy must.

(Of course, if a shark tries to eat your child, even though the shark is simply doing what it must, you know what you need to do.)

Bureaucracy should not be called evil. It *is* amorphous, ubiquitous, nameless, and faceless. It's so insidious that it hides from us. That's what makes it sly, underhanded and potentially lethal.

It is comforting to point the finger of blame at some*one* and not some*thing*. It feels good when you can look at some prominent fat cat—corporate or political—and say, "That's who's to blame for all my woes." It does not satisfy at all to say the villain is the amorphous, nameless, and faceless bureaucracy. Yet, it is the true culprit.

Bureaucracy is massive—the healthcare bureaucracy overwhelmingly so. In fact, healthcare is the largest line item on the U.S. federal budget, and most State budgets too. As I pointed out earlier in the book, there are over six million people in the U.S. licensed to provide medical care in some form (the doers). There are over ten million[9] who "manage" those six million. These ten million are the bureaucrats.

Without a doubt, the bureaucracy is powerful. However, contrary to accepted wisdom, it is not *all*-powerful. It derives its power from us. We give it to elected officials and they, acting on orders from the cancer, tell the bureaucrats what to do. If we want the bureaucracy to change, all we have to do is say so, with our votes.

A cancer of bureaucratic greed is the root cause of sickness in U.S. healthcare. It is our ultimate enemy. The cancer is the insidious, nameless and faceless, huge and powerful villain who is dragging our healthcare system (and us with it) into an early grave.

Sun Tzu wrote in his famous *Art of War,* "Know your enemy." The winning general understands that it is not simply the enemy combatant right in front of him with sword in hand who is the enemy. It is not even the whole army arrayed against him. The ultimate enemy is the principle that mobilized that army: Conquest.

The good doctor knows that a cell in a colon cancer is merely a single soldier. What is killing the patient is the principle behind the entire cancer: Growth without limit.

When government bureaucracies started in China several thousand years ago, the bureaucrats were servants. They were the interface between the rulers and the peasants, serving both. In modern times, the servant has become our cruel master, controlling both rulers (politicians) and peasants (We The People) alike. In fact, "controlling" does not fully capture what is happening. In its drive to grow, bureaucracy is literally consuming the people it is supposed to serve.

That is precisely the problem with bureaucratic greed. It grows without any constraint and without any thought or care about what its growth will do to others. What you see are people whose decisions and actions are harming us. It is not just one political party that is to blame. Bureaucracy has co-opted both. It doesn't care whether you are Republican or Democrat. It is an "equal opportunity" devourer.

Whichever way you lean politically, the cancer of bureaucratic greed-for-growth has a tactic that works. If you are archconservative, there is a "ratchet effect," that says government expansion, once it is in place, is virtually impossible to reverse.[10] Hard core liberals believe that

Americans never give up a promised entitlement even if they don't get what was promised. Thus, the entitlement bureaucracy seems effectively immortal. Either way, bureaucracy wins. It stays in control because you and I keep going along with either the conservative ratchet effect or the liberal entitlement philosophy.

To take back control of your health care, you must ask yourself, "Am I correct to conclude that bureaucratic greed is our true, common enemy—the root cause of problems? You review the evidence. You consider the various opinions and analyses. You think for yourself, you conclude, and you *choose*.

Choose!

The final step in this process is the step we began with: Choice. Now that you have valid (not false) and complete information, you must choose. Good or bad, right or wrong, you must make a choice. You can be free or you can be entitled. You cannot be both. If you give up your freedom for a "free" anything—healthcare, a computer, or a car—it will turn out badly.

If you do not choose, that means you "sit on the fence." This plays out when you think, "oh, but some people need free healthcare." Or "I need the government to help me." But here's the catch. If you stay "on the fence," then you *choose* to give away your freedom.

A free person chooses. If you reject your ability, in fact your obligation, to decide; if you give up your power to choose to another, you enslave yourself to him or her. Yes, people actually do that, for one of three reasons: the Siren Song, victim status, and futility.

In Greek mythology, the Sirens were thought to be beautiful women who sat on the shores of the Mediterranean. They sang such sweet songs that passing boats could not resist sailing toward them into rocky shoals that would crush the boats and kill the sailors.

The "Siren Song" has come to mean a compelling, seductive message that you cannot resist. I've already alluded to this above. In healthcare, the Sirens tempt us with "free" medical care, whenever you want it, and whatever you want. The cancer is singing, "Just turn over your power, your vote, your will, your freedom, to me and I will provide all of your health care." You must resist the Sirens. Deny those who call you (or make you) a "victim."

The cancer of greed wants victims because victims enslave themselves. A victim is an individual who blames someone else for his or her lot in life. The second you accept "victim" status, you give over your right to choose—your freedom—to someone else. The solution to your problems is then in someone else's hands, not in yours. And when that someone, let's call it government bureaucracy, doesn't solve your problems, when you remain jobless living in a one-room walk-up, this just "proves" that you were right to call yourself a victim.

The upshot of that whole scenario is not pretty. If you continue to rely on the bureaucracy to fix healthcare, it's never going to be "fixed" in a way that benefits you.

If you have not heard Dr. Ben Carson's comments on being a victim, you need to take the time (twenty-seven minutes[11]) to listen to a man who went from the worst poverty in the urban housing projects to become Chief of Pediatric Neurosurgery at Johns Hopkins. He says his mother demanded that he and his brother would never, ever accept victim status.

Victims are beholden to the government because it promises to give them what they should have had but were denied. Those who claim victim status think as follows: We are entitled, but since we did not get our entitlement, or not enough of it, we are therefore *victim*, and we expect the government to make it up to us. In return, we turn over our right to choose to the government (which is really under the control of the bureaucracy.)

The third reason why people deny their freedom is something that T.J. Mullaney's calls the "consensus of futility." It's the idea that whatever you do, no matter how hard you fight, the outcome is inevitable. If that is so, why waste your time and energy? It's what the Borg in *Star Trek, The Next Generation* TV series repeated in a emotionless monotone, "Resistance is futile."

Journalist Bill Moyers bemoans what he calls "learned helplessness," referring to people who are repeatedly told that attempts at self-improvement are doomed to failure. They hear this both from those sharing their poverty as well as politicians and bureaucrats who want to control them. Those who learn to be helpless then join what reporter T.J. Mullaney called a "consensus of futility." (see cit. #383.)

You must not, repeat must not, join this consensus. If you do, you will create a *self-fulfilling prophecy*. "It can't be fixed, so I won't try," guarantees that "it" (whatever it is) will never be fixed. You have not only correctly predicted the future, but you have assured that your future will be one you don't want!

And above all, don't think that you don't have enough information or enough wisdom to make the right choice.[12] Once you take a good hard look at the ever-expanding cancer of bureaucracy growing in our government, and you will wise up to what is killing us.

Wisdom helps us choose among various options. Wisdom is necessary to prioritize our choices. It is easy to choose between good and bad. However, at other times, you must choose between good and good. The part that requires wisdom is deciding which one is good-er. This happened in a meeting a few years ago:

> Fred H. was the CEO of a large urban hospital. One day while discussing the budget, he abruptly lost focus and developed a glassy-eyed appearance. He was suddenly paying no attention. Several of us doctors began to worry he was having a stroke or a seizure.
>
> Though the silence lasted only about thirty seconds, it was painful and scary. Fred then came back to us and began musing.
>
> "Do you realize that we are sitting here talking about cutting two good, important medical services in order to keep whichever we think is the 'more needed' service. The problem is, they are **all** programs that help the patients. So when we cut, we are hurting the very people we are trying to help."
>
> Someone responded, "True, but we have to decide in the name of the greatest good for the greatest number of people."

Fred nodded in agreement but then added, "Well, I signed up to manage things in the broad sense but you doctors, you signed up to help patients one at a time. How do you cope with doing things that you know will hurt your own, individual patients who have names, feelings, families, and mortgages?"

No one replied. No one had enough wisdom to offer a good answer.

But here's an alternate and far better ending to that story. The people in that room may not have had the wisdom to offer a decent answer, but you do! Who do you think has the appropriate wisdom to make life-and-death decisions for you or for your children? Your doctor? Your insurance agent? Maybe the Medical Director of your insurance plan? Some self-styled expert or panel of experts? The Director of Medicare or the Secretary of Health and Human Services? The President? Me?

You know the answer. The best decision maker for you—I believe the only proper decision maker for you—is YOU. It is more frightening and more dangerous to let someone else make your choices for you than for you to decide.

The right decision maker for you is You. The right decision maker for healthcare is us—We The Patients.

If we want healthcare to work for our benefit and not the cancer's, then let's make it so.

Beyond Healthcare

The Fourth of July is a holy holiday. I was finishing the first edition of this book July 4, 2013. I'm finishing this, the second edition, on July 4, 2015. I can't help but reflect. No one who proudly calls himself or herself an American can ignore the significance of that day, as well as the history that led up to it.

On the Fourth, the most difficult decision most of us have to make is, which hot dog: Nathan's, Best's, Hebrew National, or Oscar Meyer? We do not give a moment's brain sweat to the price that was paid for our freedom to choose. Thomas Paine wrote, "Those who expect to reap the blessings of freedom must, like men, undergo the fatigue of supporting it."[13] Most of us just take our unlimited ability to make choices for granted and ask someone to, "Please pass the mustard."

We must never take freedom for granted. We must always keep in mind how we are free to choose and how responsibility comes with that freedom. We should pay homage to those courageous men and women of two hundred and thirty-nine years ago: what they thought, wrote, did, risked, and sometimes died for.

Patrick Henry—of "Give me liberty or give me death" fame—said, "The constitution is not an instrument for the government to restrain the people; it is an instrument for the people to restrain the government."

It appears to more and more Americans that We The People work for the government, not the other way around, not the way it should be. We do not control the government: it controls us. The cancer has invaded the bureaucracy, and commands it to grow, no matter the cost. The ever-growing bureaucracy dictates to the government, and we suffer. The tail is wagging the dog.[14]

To be faithful to the principles on which our country was founded, we cannot give up our right to choose and the responsibility that comes with it. Why would we even *think* of trading away our most precious possession—freedom—for empty promises such as free healthcare or impossible entitlements based on income "redistribution?"[15]

The cancer has not limited itself to healthcare. It has metastasized to all aspects of government. The cancer spurs the government bureaucracy to get bigger and bigger. It thrives and grows as we bleed to death.

The bureaucracy eats dollars that we desperately need for schools, road repairs, raising the levees around New Orleans, or paying our doctors. Meanwhile, thousands of federal regulators and IRS agents have shiny new jobs, even as two of my neighbors go on unemployment. Our Representatives exempt themselves from a law—ACA—they passed, saying it was good for the American people. If it is so good for us, why is it not good for them?

The government controls us with the "promise them anything" tactic. We cannot say we weren't warned. In 1787, Alexander Tyler, a Scottish history professor, wrote, "A democracy will continue to exist up until the time that voters discover they can vote themselves generous gifts from the public treasury. From that moment on, the majority always votes for the candidates who promise the most benefits from the public treasury."

Buying our votes with high-sounding rhetoric and empty promises is a strategy that works, but only as long as we let it.[16] It succeeds only while as we keep our eyes shut and our minds turned off, depend on "hope," ignore the evidence, and leave the cancer alone.

Imagine if we applied what I have outlined in this chapter—look past the disinformation and think for yourself—not only to healthcare, but to all aspects of our government and society? Might it be possible that we could actually turn the cancer of greed to our advantage and simultaneously retake control of our country and ourselves? That is what we want. That is what we need. That is what I hope you choose to do.

God bless America, especially the principles for which, and on which, it stands. It is a return to those principles that will show us the way to take back control and restore the American healthcare system to where it should be.

Finally, thinking is vital, necessary, indeed critical to correct decision-making, but it is not enough. We must take action. After we think for ourselves and decide what is true and what is not, what should we *do*?

ELEVEN

Take Back Control Of Healthcare

To cure a patient, a good doctor treats the cause of the patient's illness. A proper doctor does not treat symptoms alone and does not say that painkillers are a cure. An ethical doctor never, ever, ever, EVER forces a harmful treatment down an unwilling patient's throat.

I have spent this entire book diagnosing the cause of sickness in the American healthcare system. Healthcare is the patient. The diagnosis is cancer, cancer of the bureaucracy.

As noted in the introduction, bureaucracy is a necessary, vital part of any organization, industry, or society. A doctor cannot simply cut out bureaucracy and expect a system to survive. Just as a surgeon needs to do with any vital organ in the human body, we must keep the bureaucracy alive while killing the cancer.

The difference between a healthy cell and a cancer cell is control. Your body controls the healthy cells. It does not control malignant cells, and therefore, the body cannot stop the cancer cells from over-growing. A body is cancer-free when it has taken back control of all its cells. The cure for the cancer in healthcare's bureaucracy is to regain control.

To save patient Healthcare and ourselves at the same time, we must restore OUR control of healthcare, taking control away from cancer that has taken over Washington.

In preparation for this book, we did several surveys of average Americans about healthcare. For every question except one, we received differing opinions and various viewpoints.

On one question, there was one hundred percent agreement. Regardless of age, gender, economic status, education level, or political affiliation, when asked, "Who should control your health care," every respondent without exception vehemently answered, "Me, and no one else!"

The saying below should become our slogan.

WASHINGTON – Don't Control Me!!

Direct-Pay USA = I Control Me

The "Post Obamacare" in the book's title is a *double entendre*, French for two distinctly different meanings for the same word or phrase.

One meaning of Post could be "after implementation" of the Affordable Care Act. Starting January 1, 2014, we have evidence-of-effect, not prognostications, rosy or dire. We no longer have to depend on neither the Democrats' wish fulfillment promises nor the Republicans' warnings of the apocalypse to come. That is what you just read in chapter 10.

A second meaning for "Post" is without Obamacare, after Obamacare is gone. What might such a Post Obamacare world look like? Might patient Healthcare remain critically ill or even die?

One of Republicans' war cries for the past five years has been Repeal and Replace. They have never suggested precisely *what* they would replace Obamacare with. To them and to you, I offer Direct-Pay USA. This would be a Post Obamacare world where healthcare does what it should and is healthy.

Several years ago, some courageous doctors began to say, "We no longer accept insurance. Just pay us a flat fee in cash." This became known as concierge medicine.[1] As this was very expensive, only the extremely wealthy could afford it. If you ever watched the TV series called *Royal Pains*, you will note that a show featuring a concierge doctor took place in the New York Hamptons, one of the wealthiest communities in the nation.

The idea of a return to direct doctor-patient financial as well as medical relationship is catching on and not just for Hampton-dwellers. The idea of "direct-pay" medicine is exemplified by the Oklahoma Surgical Center. These doctors only accept cash-out-of-pocket as payment for their services. They openly publish all-inclusive prices as well as their risk-adjusted medical outcomes. The patient knows exactly what he or she is buying.

Direct-pay practices also negotiate prices with suppliers such as labs or x-ray services for a cash-on-the-barrelhead, best price for their patients. The usual bill sent to insurance for a lipid panel (cholesterol and triglycerides) is $90. Direct-pay patients pay $5, in cash, directly to the lab. No paper work. No forms to fill out. No review process. No waiting for a year to get reimbursed.

A few months ago, I was on a local radio talk show. During the first half, the host interviewed me. The second half was devoted to people calling in with questions or comments. One woman told her direct-pay history, which I share here.

The caller was a veteran. She had severe back problems (not war injuries) that required major spine surgery. She was in constant pain and unable to walk. When she called our local VA hospital, they said she was covered. They could schedule the operation in about a year. Insurance would pay much but not all of the $126,000 price tag. She said thank you and hung up.

She began searching and shopping on the Internet. She found the facility in Oklahoma and reviewed their results for the surgery that she needed as well as their price: $11,250, cash. Even over the phone, you could hear the smile on her face. She concluded by reporting she is pain free and starting to jog again.

A number of medical practices are turning to a no-insurance, direct-pay model.[2] Doctors in these practices recommend their patients get a stop-loss, or catastrophic health insurance policy that pays for everything after a very large deductible, say $10,000.

The patients are happy. Direct-pay doctors are ecstatic. They are making roughly the same income as they did when they took insurance and certainly before ACA. They have better relationships with their patients because they can spend the time necessary to talk to their patients and simply be with them. Best of all, the hassle factor is almost gone.[3]

In an earlier book titled *Uproot U.S. Healthcare*, I describe a root cause of healthcare's woes as "micro-economic disconnection." Our third party payment system disconnects demand (patient) from supply (doctor). This eliminates any of our powerful, consumer-friendly free market forces. It also severs the fiduciary connection between doctor and patient. Direct-pay medicine restores that connection and the free market forces that come with it.

In the story of the woman veteran, I hope you noticed the effect on your wallet of direct-pay. Medical care suddenly becomes affordable when the government is removed from healthcare, and free market forces are allowed to work. Consumers will spend wisely (it's *their* own money) and sellers will compete for consumers' dollars both on price and results.

For many years, Washington has used fraud-and-abuse within Medicare as a whipping boy to divert our attention from how many of our dollars federal BARRC (chapter seven) was wasting. They crow about the tens of billions they recover by prosecuting fraud-and-abuse so we won't notice the trillions they spend on themselves, wasting money on useless bureaucracy that is desperately needed for patient services. Consider billing and coding.

This is the process where the provider hires a biller to fill out the proper forms and a coder adds the correct 5-digit code numbers that relate to what the doctor and hospital did for you. These forms go to insurance companies and then the federal government for verification; putting the information into a huge database; and eventually, the providers get paid whatever the federal reimbursement allows for the codes specified.

Billing and coding is one of the largest departments in any hospital. They not only do the billing and coding, but they try to keep up with the constant changes in the rules so that the institution will not be (please God, no!) Out of Compliance. Their Department is a very large expense item on every bottom line.

Keep in mind that all Medicare fraud-and-abuse occurs within the billing process. Examples of such fraud-and-abuse include:

- Up-coding: using a code that pays more rather than the code for what was actually done.
- Phantom billing: submitting bills for services that weren't performed or for patients who do not exist
- Double billing: sending in two bills for one service.
- Errors: given the complexity and ever-changing rules and regulations, honest errors are bound to occur yet they are considered fraud and abuse.

Many years ago, a whistle blower reported to Washington that Children's Hospital of Philadelphia was double billing. This great institution was reputably submitting bills for services from both the Attending (teaching) physician and the Resident doctor (in training). Even though this was (and still is) standard practice, the hospital quickly settled for $20 million. The last thing they wanted was to anger the 800-pound gorilla (and their biggest payer by far) called the federal government. The whistle blower got 10 percent.

Now envision a world where there is no billing and coding. No more Medicare fraud-and-abuse! No more wasteful spending on useless bureaucracy. Think of the money we could save! Health care becomes cheaper. As an added bonus, you get a bill from the doctor or hospital with simple words not meaningless numbers (codes).

THAT is the world of Direct-Pay USA. The doctor bills the patient. The patient pays the doctor. No billers or coders in between to confuse things and then take "just a small piece" of the action.

Suppose everyone in America had his or her own HSA (Health Savings Account) and it could build it up over decades without limit. Suddenly, the woman veteran above could shell out $11,250 without breaking a sweat. The 70-year old who needs cancer treatment costing $150,000 would not have a heart attack thinking about paying for what he needs.

Dr. Ben Carson advocated such a concept at a National Prayer Breakfast on February 13, 2013.[4] That speech launched him to national prominence and sparked widespread interest in his running for the White House in 2016.

We do not have to actively kill the cancer in our healthcare system. We can simply let it wither away from non-use. Give Americans the choice between Obamacare and Direct-Pay USA. Watch what happens.

Direct-Pay USA is simple, as any good plan should be. It is the opposite of complex. Patients *decide* and patients *pay for* their health care choosing among competing doctors, hospitals, and services. Where does the money come from? Answer: every year, the government puts $5000 into Health Savings Accounts for every American, each and every one of 320 million people. That money can accumulate over time but can only be used for medical care. The money comes from tax revenues, but before you have a stroke thinking that is *additional, new* spending, read on in the Economics section below to see how it actually saves money.

Medicare eligible individuals will receive a payout into their HSAs of the amount they contributed over their working lifetime. This will mean over a hundred thousand dollars for each person over sixty-five years of age.

No more incomprehensible insurance forms. No more government telling your doctor what she or he cannot do for you. No more denials. No more over-spending on healthcare.

Economics of Direct-Pay USA

In late 2014, Deloitte Consultants released a report[5] on how much the U.S. actually spent on healthcare in 2012. As a nation we spent $3.4 trillion. Our population was then almost 313 million.

Our present population is 320 million. If the government put $5000 into 320 million HSAs, that would cost $1.6 trillion for healthcare, which is less than half (!) what we spent on healthcare in 2012, *before* Obamacare was implemented.

I know the first thought in your mind when I say, "pay for your own care" is, "It's too expensive. I cannot possibly afford $15,000 for a hernia repair much less half a million for chemotherapy." As you will see, these concerns melt away with Direct-Pay.

The prices or charges (no one knows true costs) for healthcare goods and services at present are not subjected to free market competition. You saw what happened when the government was cut out of the equation and free market restored in the veteran example above that I learned during a call-in radio show. Suddenly, you can get your hernia repair for $1500 or $2000, readily affordable amounts from an HSA containing, say, $20,000 or $30,000.

Note also that when you pay for your own care, you can decide who should operate, i.e., where and with whom you can get the best results for the best dollar value.

Also note that even a $15,000 charge will not frighten you when you have saved your $5000 per year for five years of good health and your account reads: "$25,000 available for medical care for _____ (fill in your name)."

Finally, let me shock you with what you actually spent on healthcare in 2012. You may not know you are paying this because the money is taken out your wallet through hidden taxes on individuals, companies, and organizations. The math is simple, real, compelling, and outrageous.

What YOU spent on Healthcare in 2012:

U.S. spent: $3,400,000,000,000
> divided by

U.S. population: 312,780,968

> equals: **$10,870**

What you actually spent in 2012 was $10,870, yes, over ten thousand, just for you. You spent another $10,870 for your spouse, and again $10,870 for each of your two children. The average family of four, without knowing and *without their consent*, thus spent $43,480 on healthcare in 2012.

I can hear you exclaiming, "That's impossible! No one can pay $43,480 into the healthcare system when the median income for a U.S. household is only $51,939." Let me reassure you. That $43,480 is an average across 312 million people. For every one person who paid a million dollars, there were twenty-three people who paid nothing. And remember, most of that spending is new dollar bills printed just for Obamacare and paid not by you or me, but to be paid by our grandchildren, as it is added to the national debt.

Direct-Pay would eliminate that massive, hidden withdrawal from your bank account made by the cancer. And if we all chose to use the Direct-Pay model, Obamacare would soon become a painful but distant memory.

While a number of details must be worked out, here are the answers to some obvious questions.

What about access to care for the poor? Answer: Even those with no income at all would quickly have tens of thousands of dollars in their HSAs to spend on health care needs.

What about insurance? I personally believe stop-loss insurance should be built into Direct-Pay USA. People would buy catastrophic insurance, which would pay for everything after the patient spends some upper limit out of the HSA, say, $10,000. This certainly should be debated, and decided, by us.

How should illegal residents be handled under Direct-Pay? Many illegals are tax-paying members of society. Yet they are ineligible for government-supported insurance. I suggest that they receive the same $5000 per year as everyone else. Then like everyone else, they pay for the care they receive, and buy insurance.

Others may feel differently and that's fine. What should happen is open discussion and debate followed by a decision made by We The People about the financing of the health care of American non-citizens. What should *not* happen is what Washington is doing now—avoiding the issue. Policy for illegal residents should not be left buried like some dark secret and ignored because politicians are too fearful of polarization to have an open dialogue.

Wouldn't the Direct-Pay Plan put tens of thousands of healthcare bureaucrats out of work: Actuaries, lawyers, billers and coders, regulators, and compliance officers to name a few? Answer: yes. I do not want to pay for them and neither do you.

Are there are issues to be discussed and decided by us? Certainly. However, Direct-Pay USA would begin the process of curing the cancer that is currently killing patient Healthcare.

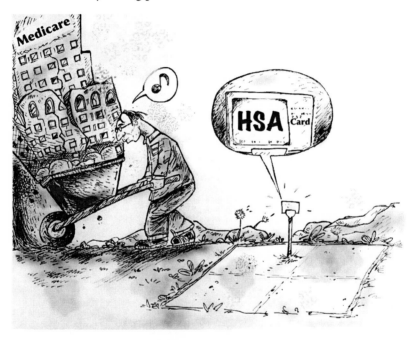

Most will love it. Progressives won't.

Most Americans are what I call "social liberals" (not socialist). Like me, they believe there should be a medical safety net so that everyone, rich and poor alike, can get the care they need.

If you are a conservative, you will love this plan because it is restores personal responsibility to healthcare.

The culture of the U.S. will applaud Direct-Pay USA as it enshrines our most sacred value: independence—personal liberty.

Ardent defenders of the Constitution understand that Direct-Pay is precisely what the Framers would want. In fact, it was the system that the five physicians who signed the Declaration of Independence worked in.

Forty-three percent of Americans who pay no federal taxes could be called the poor.[6] The poor will love this plan because they will be able to get insurance just like everyone else; and with cash in hand, they will have ready access to care, which they do not have now.

We The Patients are sure to love Direct-Pay as it *gets the government out* of the doctor's office and out of their wallets.

Progressives won't like this cure for healthcare at all. Progressives believe that they know what is best for people, better than the people do themselves. Progressives control your money and your health care decisions because they believe they can do a better job than you can. "It is for your own good, Trust me!" they shout. Since Direct-Pay takes control from them and returns it to you, progressives won't like it.

The Federal bureaucracy, firmly under the control of cancer, is sure to push back because of all the jobs (and votes) they will lose.

Some Washington politicians will love this proposal and some will hate it. Those who want to keep working for the cancer will oppose Direct-Pay USA. Those who wish to return to doing the jobs they were elected to do will embrace it.

Are You A "Greater Fool?"

The first step to fix healthcare is to take off the rose-colored glasses. **There is no quick, simple, easy, cheap, painless cure** for Healthcare. Anyone who says such a thing exists is (a) living with Alice in Wonderland; (b) a magical thinker; c) running for re-election; or (d) an expert consultant like Jonathan Gruber who is selling his own particular brand of snake oil for an exorbitant price.[7] Don't buy it. You know better. You certainly should by now.

Doctors say that the first step in healing is to accept that you are sick, that you are a *patient*. For patient Healthcare, there is a second "first step."

After accepting that Healthcare is sick, We The Patients—you and me down in the trenches—must accept that we are the *doctors* for

Healthcare. If we are waiting for Washington to fix healthcare, we are expecting cancer to cure cancer. Never happen.

The hardest step is mental. We must **know** that we can do it.

I frequently hear people say, "I'm just one person. What can I do against the power of the government?" or, "There must be someone else better than me. Let him (or her) fix it." Can you imagine George Washington, Thomas Jefferson, or Patrick Henry saying those things?

The HBO TV series *The Newsroom* is one of my favorites. From one of the episodes, I learned what I am. I am a "greater fool."

A greater fool is someone whom others see as impractical, illogical, and foolish, someone who doesn't accept life's "obvious" limitations.

On *The Newsroom*, Sloan is the expert in Economics. She described the greater fool as the person "we toss the hot potato to; we dive for his seat when the music stops. The greater fool is someone with the perfect blend of self-delusion and ego to think that he can succeed where others have failed."[8]

The greater fool finds a way to do what others say can't be done. This fool rejects the consensus of futility and its self-fulfilling prophecy. The greater fool is the dreamer who turns his impossible dreams into reality.

After a breathy pause, Sloan ends the dialogue above in *The Newsroom* by softly declaring, "This whole country was *made* by greater fools."

To cure patient Healthcare and save ourselves at the same time, we need a large number of greater fools. I'm one. How about you?

Chapter Notes

Introduction

1   At the outset, we need to resolve the confusion about names. President Obama's healthcare reform law started life named House Resolution 3590. What was passed in March 2010 was called the Patient Protection and Affordable Health Care Act (PPAHCA). Detractors named it Obamacare as a pejorative, until the President said he actually liked the name. In its five years of life, the Law has been abbreviated as PPAHCA, PPACA, AHCA, and currently ACA—Affordable Care Act. For simplicity, we will consistently refer to the 2010 healthcare reform Act as the ACA or Obamacare.

2   Mr. Spock, the famous Vulcan character in the original TV show *Star Trek* (1967-69) was supposed to live life purely from a logical, emotionless perspective but displayed wonderfully human characteristics. Sadly, in 2015 we lost Leonard Nimoy, the man who played Mr. Spock on the TV series and in many subsequent movies based on that series.

Chapter 1

No notes needed

Chapter 2

1   Alexis-Charles-Henri Clérel de Tocqueville is probably best known for his two volumes (1835 & 1840) titled, *Democracy in America*.

2   After the first estimate of $780 billion of *new spending*, Washington upped their projection to $1.3 trillion and then later down to "only" $1.1 trillion. See: http://www.huffingtonpost.com/2012/03/15/health-care-reform_n_1347327.html.

3   Initially, then-House Speaker Nancy Pelosi promised grandly, that ACA would cut healthcare costs but had no supporting evidence. The initial cost projection from Washington was over $800 billion. At the same time, Kaiser Research Foundation estimated the cost at $2.7 trillion. Since the original government estimate, Washington has revised upward its spending projection to $1.76 trillion or maybe $1.3 trillion, possibly only $1.1 trillion. That is NEW SPENDING—the opposite of cost cutting. For a sense of perspective, $2.7 trillion is more than the total U.S. military expenditure for ten-plus years of War in both Iraq and Afghanistan.

4   See: http://usatoday30.usatoday.com/news/opinion/editorials/2005-02-09-edit_x.htm and http://www.democraticunderground.com/discuss/duboard.php?az=view_all&address=389x6176555.

5   See: http://blogs.wsj.com/washwire/2009/06/15/obama-if-you-like-your-doctor-you-can-keep-your-doctor.

6   See S. Fitzgerald's "Obamacare Fallout: More Doctors Opting Out of Medicare" at http://www.newsmax.com/Newsfront/Obamacare-Medicare-doctors-drop/2013/07/29/id/517497.

7   *The Hill* reported, "HHS to cut off enrollment for health law's high-risk pools," at: http://thehill.com/policy/healthcare/283557-report-hhs-to-cut-off-enrollment-for-health-laws-high-risk-pools

Chapter 3

1   See: Associated Press' "Accusation Glaxo paid Chinese doctors shines light on abuses in cash-starved medical system," at: www.washingtonpost.com/world/asia_pacific/accusation-glaxo-paid-chinese-doctors-shines-light-on-abuses-in-cash-starved-medical-system/2013/08/01/108b7ad6-fa61-11e2-89f7-8599e3f77a67_story.html.

2   Read about why our med-mal system can't possibly do what the people expect in "The U.S. Needs Tort Replacement, Not Just "Reform." It was published in several online venues including LinkedIn and the *Journal of Socialomics 2014*; 3:1-6.

3   Citation 541 in the Author Reference section is an analysis of fifty medical malpractice cases in children. It confirms that most juries do indeed make the automatic conclusion that since the death of a child is unnatural, someone must have made a medical error.

4   For any physicians reading, the baby had TGA with VSD, transposition of the great arteries with [mal-alignment] ventricular septal defect.

5   Dr. Ed Marsh wrote an Op-Ed piece in the *Wall Street Journal* (040713) explaining why he had to quit practicing medicine. He was just as unhappy about doing it as I was. Read him at: http://online.wsj.com/article/SB10001424127887324789504578380382204116270.html.

Chapter 4

1   For those individuals who may have never played Monopoly®, let me explain. It is a very popular board game where two to six players try to win by gaining control—monopoly—over the properties on the board. It was created by Parker Brothers and is now distributed by Hasbro Toy Company.

2   Numerous online and newspaper articles described the plight of this unfortunate boy. Fingers were pointed at everyone except the real culprit: the cancer of greed. See: http://abcnews.go.com/Health/Dental/story?id =2925584&page=1#.UMUCxb90oUI.

3   See: http://fdlaction.firedoglake.com/2013/04/30/actually-obama-your-health-care-law-will-not-stop-medical-bankruptcy, and http://content.healthaffairs.org/content/25/2/w89.long.

4   To view my source data, go to: http://www.ncsl.org/issues-research/health/health-insurance-premiums.aspx. You can even see the State-by-State costs: they vary considerably.

5   See "Obamacare Premiums Increased Dramatically for Every Age Group in 2014," by JR. Graham, October 30, 2014 at: http://healthblog.ncpa.org/obamacare-premiums-increased-dramatically-for-every-age-group-in-2014

6   See articles by Harold Mandel at: http://www.examiner.com/article/study-shows-millions-of-americans-are-without-adequate-health-insurance and by Jon Walker at: http://fdlaction.firedoglake.com/2013/04/30/actually-obama-your-health-care-law-will-not-stop-medical-bankruptcy.

7   See: The Reason Health Care Is So Expensive: Insurance Companies, 4/10/13 by J. Pfeffer at: http://www.businessweek.com/articles/2013-04-10/the-reason-health-care-is-so-expensive-insurance-companies.

8   It is ironic that the federal government released its hold on highly dangerous prescription drugs just after it tightened advertising regulations on one of the most dangerous non-prescription, highly addictive over-the-counter drugs known, called nicotine (cigarettes).

9   President Richard Charles Levin retired in 2013 after a highly successful stint of more than twenty years. He was replaced by the Provost, Peter Salovey.

10   The quote comes, of course from possibly the greatest of Shakespeare's plays, Hamlet, who said, "Therein lies the rub, For in that sleep of death we know not what dreams may come...." Maybe Hamlet's thoughts of suicide were caused one of those anti-depression or anti-arthritis drugs that they advertise on TV.

Chapter 5

1 My son lives in Turkey, which has a Constitution and rule of law, yet President Erdoğan is able attack his political enemies with the power of the government. When I read about what the IRS got away with when it selectively targeted political groups opposed to President Obama, I begin to fear for our great nation. To date, no one has been brought to justice for these illegal acts.

2 It is downright frightening to watch the Washington bureaucratic machinery—IRS, OCEA, ATF, INS—become a tool of political coercion and silencing of political dissent under the Obama Administration. Former IRS Director Lois Lerner got away with destroying evidence when she "lost" emails that would have proven federal malfeasance. Hillary Clinton seems to have gotten away by using the same ploy. For a real eye-opener, watch businesswoman and founder of True The Vote, Katherine Englebrecht testify before Congress. Access: http:// www.realclearpolitics.com/video/2014/02/06/true_the_vote_found-er_to_congress_i_will_not_retreat_i_will_not_surrender_i_refuse_to_be_intimidated.html. You will no doubt ask, what resulted from her eloquent plea for decency and honesty in government? Answer: nothing.

3 The whole concept of an unlimited health care entitlement is being called into question in Great Britain, where some fear the entire NHS will collapse. See: http://rt.com/news/uk-nhs-health-crisis-049.

4 The Flemming v. Nestor case involved Social Security not Medicare (which had not been created in 1960). Ephram Nestor was deported for being a Communist. The government terminated his Social Security benefits under Section 202(n) of the Social Security Act. Nestor sued to get his payments claiming he had a contract with the government. The Supreme Court held that no such contract existed and that Nestor's payments into Social Security were not his "property," and thus were not protected under the Fifth Amendment to the Constitution, the famous "Takings" clause.

5 See: http://www.garynorth.com/public/7789.cfm and http:// www.forbes.com/sites/merrillmatthews/2012/08/21/ think-social-securitys-trust-fund-is-a-scam-medicare-has-one-too.

6 For explanation of what MACRA is and why is won't solve Medicare's problems, see: http://www.theblaze.com/contributions/ for-medicare-another-fix-that-fails

7 See citations 28 and 305 as well as, "Why Medicaid is a Humanitarian Catastrophe by Avik Roy, at: http://www.forbes.com/sites/ aroy/2011/03/02/why-medicaid-is-a-humanitarian-catastrophe.

8   Reported as "Nearly A Third Of Doctors Won't See New Medicaid Patients," Aug 06, 2012 at: http://www.kaiserhealthnews.org/ Stories/2012/August/06/Third-Of-Medicaid-Doctors-Say-No-New-Patients.aspx.

9   The issue of government intrusiveness into our private lives is becoming a bigger and bigger concern. First there were invasions of Associated Press source information sources, and then came the matter of federal blanket (not targeted) acquisition of Verizon telephone records. And of course, I only need these three letters to get your attention: NSA. "Big Brother" apparently really IS watching you.

10   George Orwell's novel *1984* described a totalitarian government that controlled everything, including our thoughts and punished that which was not government-approved. It was written in 1948, when the reality of the Communist total control was becoming evident to the whole world. Health care providers today see the constant expansion of federal rules and regulations as taking over control of doctors and nurses. In the book *1984*, the slogan touted everywhere was, "Big Brother is watching you."

11   Look at a graph of Congressional approval and be astonished how low it goes. If more than 80% of your employees did a bad job, why would you keep them? See: http://www.realclearpolitics.com/epolls/other/congressional_job_approval-903.html.

12   Aldous Huxley's book, *Brave New World* was written in 1931, seventeen years before *1984*. Though Huxley's book is often compared with Orwell's *1984*, they are very different. Where Orwell feared that the government would conceal the truth from us, Huxley feared the truth would be drowned in a sea of irrelevant data and manufactured opinion. What do you think? I fear both authors were right.

13   Us 'old folks' know, because we have experienced so much of life, the wisdom of the phrase, "It is better to ask for forgiveness than permission."

14   A Black Hole is a place in space where light goes in but cannot escape. Gravity is generated by mass. More mass=more gravity. A sufficiently dense mass, such as a collapsed star, can create such extreme gravitational pull that even photons of light cannot escape. That is why it is called a "black" (no light) hole.

15 The evidence shows clearly that the NHS does not work to the benefit of the people and is in fact failing both medically and financially. See: http://rt.com/news/hospital-cover-up-uk-190; http://frontpagemag. com/2012/dgreenfield/government-health-care-kills-more-brits-than-guns-kill-americans; http://americanthinker.com/2014/09/in_the_toi-let__british_nhs_today_us_healthcare_tomorrow.html; http://www. telegraph.co.uk/health/healthnews/9639090/Cystic-Fibrosis-sufferer-denied-chance-of-life-drug-by-NHS.html; http://www.mailtribune. com/apps/pbcs.dll/article?AID=/20120811/OPINION/208110306/-1/ NEWSMAP; and http://www.independent.co.uk/life-style/ health-and-families/health-news/nhs-reforms-hospitals-under-pres-sure-2265782.html.

16 I have warned several times (as have others) about what happens when the government budget literally decrees your life or your death. See: http://www.americanthinker.com/2011/12/actually_health_care_costs_ are_under_control.html; and particularly, "Cutting costs by killing patients," at: http://www.americanthinker.com/2013/02/cutting_health-care_costs_by_killing_patients.html

Chapter 6

1 The quote came from Lawrence Fedewa, a reporter for the *Washington Times*. See: www.washingtontimes.com/news/2014/jul/3/ fedewa-bureaucracy-fourth-branch-government/?page=all

2 It has been known for many years that patients after a transplant are more prone to develop cancers in many places in addition to the trans-planted organ. The reason is this: Drugs needed to prevent rejection suppress the entire immune system. So when some cancer cells start to grow (anywhere), the immune system doesn't work, can't kill them, and the cancer can take hold.

3 You may recall the scandal during the Iraq war when it was reported that U.S. "armored vehicles" lacked the right type of armor to protect our troops. See: http://www.washingtonpost.com/wp-dyn/content/ article/2007/02/11/AR2007021101345.html Ask yourself why did that happen and then check out the number of boxes in the organizational bureaucracy chart with names of bureaucrats who must be paid. Note the absence of a single soldier's name.

4 Various estimates have been suggested for the cost of the president's healthcare reform Act, ranging from $900 billion to $2.6 trillion, which is equal to the entire GDP of France. See: http://www.weeklystandard. com/blogs/obamacare-now-estimated-cost-26-trillion-first-de-cade_648413.html

5   See Steffie Woolhandler's article in the *New England Journal of Medicine,* 2003; 349:768-775, "The Cost of Healthcare Administration in the United States and Canada."

6   See: *The Beacon Blog.* The Independent Institute. "The Federal Bureaucracy-Plutocracy," at: http://blog.independent.org/2009/12/12/the-federal-bureaucracy-plutocracy

7   The perfect example is the King v. Burwell case described in chapter 9.

8   The first estimate for build-out of healthcare.gov was $300 million. Later it was $834 million but a more reliable, *non-government* calculation suggests a cost of $2.1 billion. See: http://www.nationalreview.com/corner/389187/how-much-did-healthcaregov-really-cost-more-administration-tells-us-veronique-de-rugy

9   This 1788 quote comes from James Madison's Federalist paper #51, which he wrote twenty years before he became President.

10 Penny Starr reported the page length in the Federal Register on CNS News at: http://cnsnews.com/news/article/penny-starr/obamacare-regulations-are-8-times-longer-bible.

11 See Chris Jacobs' article: "The IRS and Obamacare," June 5, 2013. *The Foundry.* http://blog.heritage.org/2013/06/05/the-irs-and-obamacare-by-the-numbers and at www.heritage.org

12 As this book goes to press, the number of major changes in the ACA stands at 54 (see: http://www.forbes.com/sites/gracemarieturner/2015/07/01/54-changes-to-obamacare-latest-additions/?mc_cid=96465ce41a&mc_eid=4f671091a3). Thirty-four of these changes were made without the proper statutory authority. Don't forget the tens of thousands of rule changes in addition to the major alterations described.

13 The egregious injustice of penalizing an employer who tries to provide for an employee's insurance is not found in the ACA. It was simply "pronounced" by the IRS. See: "What changes to Obamacare could mean for small-business taxes," at: http://www.marketwatch.com/story/what-changes-to-obamacare-could-mean-for-small-business-taxes-2015-06-16?mc_cid=289d1b107a&mc_eid=4f671091a3

Chapter 7

1   Fabio Casartelli was not the first cyclist to die during the Tour de France, just the first to die from a crash. Tommy Simpson, former World Champion, died during the 1967 Tour de France. He tried to enhance his performance with amphetamines and then added alcohol to the mix. He collapsed and died during the hotly contested climb up the famous (infamous among cyclists) Mont Ventoux.

2 Nancy Pelosi's fairyland wishful thinking has been aired many times in public. On the Charlie Rose Show (https://www.youtube.com/watch?v=CsRsLf5i16c) she confidently predicted the Democrats would keep the majority in the House before the 2014 elections. On *Meet the Press* (http://www.politifact.com/truth-o-meter/statements/2012/jul/06/nancy-pelosi/nancy-pelosi-says-everybody-will-get-more-and-pay-) she really was out of touch with reality promising everyone could get more health care and pay less for it.

3 Kerr's paper (citation 276) is required reading for the MBA degree. It should also be mandatory in medical schools. Humans are human wherever they are and what Kerr wrote applies to all human beings.

4 A whole chapter in Uproot U.S. Healthcare (citation 556) is devoted to the subject of perverse incentives. In there I wrote the following. "We rarely get what we want. We never get what we deserve. We always get what we reward."

5 See: http://www.cato.org/publications/commentary/ed-cranes-hopes-fine-publication.

6 See: http://veracitystew.com/2012/07/06/tax-or-penalty-who-is-exempt-from-the-individual-mandate-chart. Muslims and Scientologists are named exempt religious groups. For union exemptions, see: http://news.heartland.org/newspaper-article/2012/03/06/labor-unions-get-lions-share-final-aca-waivers.

7 The actual payment system for the *free* care that illegal residents receive, mandated by EMTALA, is so convoluted that it should be called Byzantine. The cost of this care is literally in the hundreds of billions. No medical system can afford to provide it and simply write it off, as they would go bankrupt immediately. (In my own hospital, that cost—mandatory "spending" as far as the hospital is concerned—is roughly 20% of the entire operating budget!) This "free care" is not free at all: it is paid by over-charging insured patients, and through the Medicaid Disproportionate Share (MDS), an extra amount paid by Medicaid to those institutions, like most inner city hospitals, that provide the bulk of such care. Interestingly, The White House is planning on canceling MDS. See: http://thehill.com/blogs/regwatch/pending-regs/295821-deadline-delays-loom-over-obamacare-rule?tmpl=component. I have no idea how hospitals like mine, which depends on MDS, will survive financially.

8 Congress has made itself exempt from ACA because they are worried that their staff will not be able to afford the extra costs associated with the law. See: http://marginalrevolution.com/marginalrevolution/2013/04/will-congress-exempt-itself-from-aca.html. Wasn't ACA supposed to make insurance more affordable, not less?

9   I am *not* making this stuff up: my imagination doesn't stretch that
    far. To check out proof, see: "IRS employee union: We don't want
    Obamacare" by Joel Gehrke at: http://washingtonexaminer.com/
    irs-employee-union-we-dont-want-obamacare/article/2533520.

10 The U.S. Supreme Court struck down the "individual mandate" as
    unconstitutional. It preserved the legality of the entire ACA bill only by
    saying the penalty for not having insurance was a "tax." See: National
    Federation Of Independent Business Et Al. v. Sebelius, Secretary Of
    Health And Human Services, Et Al. No. 11-393. Argued March 26, 27,
    28, 2012—Decided June 28, 2012.

11 Grace-Marie Turner, President of the Galen Institute, posted her
    "sticker shock" calculations on the Institute's web site and in the New
    York Post at: http://www.nypost.com/p/news/opinion/opedcolumnists/
    obamacare_pain_v9diAizoMoRa8bvkShVG0J.

12 See the evidence at: http://godfatherpolitics.com/8239/
    college-cuts-staff-hours-to-avoid-obamacare-costs.

13 See: Interview with Darren M. at New Genesis, Denver Colorado. 24
    July, 2013

14 See: "Fewer Californians Get Health Care At Work" by Judy Lin at:
    http://www.insurancejournal.com/news/west/2013/04/12/288244.htm

15 See: http://www.lifehealthpro.com/2013/02/19/
    feds-close-pcip-in-23-states.

16 Kinsey's remarks can be found at: http://finance.townhall.com/
    columnists/michaelfcannon/2013/04/22/union-seeks-repeal-of-
    obamacare-n1574579. Also, see: http://www.philly.com/philly/news/
    nation_world/20130526_Unions_cool_to_health-care_law.html.

17 "The Emperor's New Clothes" is a short story by Hans Christian
    Andersen about two weavers who promise their Emperor a new suit
    of clothes that is invisible to those unfit for their positions; or, who are
    stupid or incompetent. When the Emperor parades before his subjects
    in his *new clothes,* a child cries out, "But he isn't wearing anything at
    all!"

18 I refer to Governor Bill Richardson who was proposed as President
    Obama's Secretary of Commerce but had to withdraw his nomination
    when background checks began to reveal the amount of graft and cor-
    ruption present during Richardson's tenure as Governor of New Mexico.

19 Joseph Stalin's real name was Iosif Vissarionovich Dzhugashvili. "Stalin"
    is derived from the Russian word for "steel." He was one of the original
    seven members of the Politburo that created the Bolshevik Revolution
    in 1917 and became the undisputed totalitarian leader of the U.S.S.R. in
    1922. Stalin is considered the greatest mass murderer in history through
    his collectivization policies and later purges of political opposition.

20 "Veteran" refers to an age category (over thirty-five years old) rather than having served in the armed forces.

21 Dr. Atul Gawander, a surgeon in Boston, documented this bizarre experience in "A Lifesaving Checklist," on December 30, 2007 at: http://www.nytimes.com/2007/12/30/opinion/30gawande.html?_r=2&oref=slogin

22 In citation #185, Dr. Gawande described the New Jersey history and experience in an excellent article in *The New Yorker*. While it is interesting reading for the Public, it should be *required reading* for health care planners.

23 You probably know Leonardo de Vinci as a great artist and sculptor. Did you know that he drew designs for a modern bicycle and even a helicopter, in the 15th century!?

24 This article by George Will is well worth reading: http://www.wctrib.com/content/commentary-when-government-fails-it-tends-expand-even-faster.

25 I answered the question: "Do Americans want Single Payer," at: http://deanewaldman.com/2014/07/17/single-payer-option

26 See: Physicians for a National Health Program, "What is Single Payer?" at: http://www.pnhp.org/facts/what-is-single-payer.

27 Dan Hogberg exploded the "Myths of Single-Payer Health Care," at: http://freemarketcure.com/singlepayermyths.php#top.

28 Heath Druzin reported in *Stars and Stripes* that, "Despite scrutiny, whistleblowers say problems persist at Phoenix VA," in October 2014 at: http://www.stripes.com/news/us/despite-scrutiny-whistleblowers-say-problems-persist-at-phoenix-va-1.306857

Chapter 8

1 The legal maxim "Justice delayed in justice denied" can be traced back to the Mishnah, written in ≈200-100 BCE.

2 Citation #33 shows the decline in med school applications. There is also, by word of mouth, a dramatic fall-off in people applying for post-graduate (post-MD) training positions.

3 See the web memo by Robert Moffitt at: http://www.heritage.org/research/reports/2010/05/obamacare-impact-on-doctors.

4 See citations #538 and #542 for my evidence.

5 "Obamacare's Health-Insurance Sticker Shock" by Matthews & Litow, Jan. 13, 2013 at: http://online.wsj.com/article/SB10001424127888732393 68045782278909681000984.html.

6 See citations 34, 40, 75, 86, 114, 160, 284, 337, and 432 along with the "Report: Hospital Waiting Lists in Canada, 2007," by the Fraser Institute; and http://www.businessinsider.com/collapse-of-greeces-health-care-system-2012-12; as well as http://latino.foxnews.com/latino/health/2012/09/01/immigrants-protest-loss-free-health-care-in-spain.

7   McNamee C. 2011. Opposition demand health care review.
    Accessed March 2011 at: http://calgary.ctv.ca/servlet/an/local/
    CTVNews/20110311/ CGY_health_care_110311/20110311/
    ?hub=CalgaryHome.
8   Bragdon and Allumbaugh published an article through the Heritage
    Foundation (#2582, July 19, 2011) titled "Health care reform in Maine
    Reversing "ObamaCare Lite.""
9   The "average cost" for health insurance is a highly complex calculation
    based on age, medical circumstance, level of deductible and co-payment
    chosen, and place of residence. The reference for the $6328 amount can
    be found at: www.americanthinker.com/2011/06/ when_will_we_ever_
    learn.html.
10 See: healthinsurance.about.com/od/healthinsurancebasics/a/cost_of_
    health_insurance.htm.
11 See citation #93 for discussion of the Pentagon's recent budgetary
    problems paying for both fighter jets and healthcare benefits.
12 Dr. Atul Gawande gave the commencement address at Harvard Med in
    2011 (cit. 186). He said, "Doctors, the world of health care I and even
    you were trained for is not the world you will practice in. Teams and
    systems provide great care. We need to be pit crews, not cowboys. Just
    as in citations 545, 556 and 584), Gawande emphasized, "Great and
    cost-effective health care in the 21st century will be delivered by teams
    using coordination and feedback enabled by user-friendly IT systems."
13 This is the title of the 2001 movie starring Russell Crowe, Jennifer
    Connelly et al. It tells the story of John Forbes Nash, Jr. who won the
    Nobel Prize despite suffering from schizophrenia. His work touches
    all of our lives, including market economics, computing, evolutionary
    biology, artificial intelligence, accounting, politics, and even military
    theory.
14 Look at both the official LCP and the articles filed about it: http://www.
    mcpcil.org.uk, http://rt.com/news/hospital-cover-up-uk-190; http://
    www.catholicherald.co.uk/news/2013/01/30/peer-calls-for-liverpool-
    care-pathway-to-be-abolished; http://www.carenotkilling.org.uk/news/
    liverpool-care-pathway, and http://frontpagemag.com/2012/dgreenfield/
    government-health-care-kills-more-brits-than-guns-kill-americans.
15 Pay special attention to the public comments at the end of: http://www.
    carenotkilling.org.uk/news/liverpool-care-pathway. The article and the
    comments contradict each other rather starkly.
16 See: http://www.doctorzebra.com/prez/z_x01death_lear_g.htm.
17 See: http://www.businessweek.com/news/2012-06-13/health-care-
    spending-to-reach-20-percent-of-u-dot-s-dot-economy-by-2021.

18 Estimates for spending by ACA have ranged from a low of $1.1 trillion to a high of $2.6 trillion in the first ten years after its passage. We need to keep in mind that the federal government is quite bad at making accurate estimates of cost. In 1965, Congress projected how much Medicare would cost, but they were off juuust a little bit. Medicare cost 854% more than they estimated!

Chapter 9

1 See his story and other Obamacare horror stories at: http://townhall.com/columnists/johnhawkins/2013/10/19/5-scandalous-obamacare-horror-stories-n1727584

2 See: http://kff.org/health-costs/issue-brief/snapshots-health-care-spending-in-the-united-states-selected-oecd-countries

3 The minimum estimate for the cost of the ACA is $1.1 trillion and the upper but more likely accurate projection is $2.7 trillion, of new spending, which must be added to the deficit. See: http://news.investors.com/ibd-editorials/031412-604400-cbo-obamacare-cost-double-obama-vow.htm. Also, see: http://www.weeklystandard.com/blogs/obamacare-now-estimated-cost-26-trillion-first-decade_648413.html

4 See: http://www.weeklystandard.com/blogs/obamacare-now-estimated-cost-26-trillion-first-decade_648413.html

5 There are entirely too many of these horror stories about Obamacare. Here are several more: http://endoftheamericandream.com/archives/10-obamacare-horror-stories-that-are-almost-too-crazy-to-believe

6 The tale from the Zero Hedge Reader and other stories can be viewed at: http://endoftheamericandream.com/archives/10-obamacare-horror-stories-that-are-almost-too-crazy-to-believe

7 The subtitle of the article reads, "Thanks to mandates that take effect in 2014, premiums in individual markets will shoot up. Some may double." See: http://online.wsj.com/article/SB10001424127887323936804578227890968100984.html.

8 The title reads, "Obamacare premiums increased dramatically in every age group in 2014," at: http://healthblog.ncpa.org/obamacare-premiums-increased-dramatically-for-every-age-group-in-2014.

9 See: http://foxnewsinsider.com/2013/11/07/how-many-americans-have-lost-their-health-insurance-under-obamacare; http://www.foxnews.com/politics/2013/08/21/employers-dropping-coverage-for-thousands-spouses-over-obamacare-costs/#ixzz2eEHma1HU; http://www.chicagotribune.com/news/sns-wp-blm-news-bc-health-insure07-20150407-story.html

10 See: http://sanfrancisco.cbslocal.com/2013/06/18/aetna-to-stop-selling-individual-health-insurance-plans-in-calif/; http://www.naturalnews.com/041397_Obamacare_health_insurance_small_businesses.html#ixzz2aUvLw18r.

11 As this book went to press, the White House was claiming that 16.4 million Americans had become newly insured. However, data from Washington has been shown to be "malleable." They often use accounting gimmicks like double-counting, counting applications as though they are sign-ups, changing eligibility rules "on the fly," etc. That is why that 16.4 million number may not be accurate.

12 Read a summary in TheBlaze at: http://www.theblaze.com/contributions/with-tax-season-approaching-obamacare-is-the-only-thing-inside-your-wallet

13 Of the many warnings articles about the "affordability" consequences of the ACA, here are two you can rely on: Matthews M, Litow ME. January 14, 2013. "ObamaCare's Health-Insurance Sticker Shock." At: http://online.wsj.com/article/SB10001424127887323936804578227890968100984.html and, Cover M. January 31, 2013. "IRS: Cheapest Obamacare Plan Will Be $20,000 Per Family" at: http://cnsnews.com/news/article/irs-cheapest-obamacare-plan-will-be-20000-family.

14 Abby Goodnough reported about Ms. Maltzman in "Before Justices Rule, Floridians Consider Life Without Health subsidies, at: www.nytimes.com/2015/03/01/us/florida-health-care-supreme-court.html?_r=0

15 Check out the map of how much insurance rates rose, by state, in the Report from the Society of Actuaries, March 2013, titled, "Cost of future newly insured under the Affordable Care Act (ACA)." You can also read a good Forbes article at: http://www.forbes.com/sites/theapothecary/2013/11/04/49-state-analysis-obamacare-to-increase-individual-market-premiums-by-avg-of-41-subsidies-flow-to-elderly/#!

16 The phrase "pocket nerve" was one I learned from my now-deceased father-in-law. I used it as the title of an entire chapter in "Uproot U.S. Healthcare." See: http://t.co/sJCkZZ3a.

17 President Obama has used the phrase "rich should pay their fair share" in several contexts, including ACA mandate/penalty/tax; adjustments in the income tax code; and debt reduction plans. Here is one: http://content.usatoday.com/communities/theoval/post/2011/07/obama-opposes-short-term-debt-deal-from-boehner/1#.UdHnfL-zOiw.

18 Josh Archambault of the Pioneer Institute for Public Policy Research in Boston provided a detailed, real-world analysis of the Cadillac tax in his "Impact of the Federal Health Law's 'Cadillac Insurance Tax' in Massachusetts," October 2012.

19   See the Employee Benefits News at: http://ebn.benefitnews.com/
     news/100-dollar-day-penalties-ppaca-non-compliance-expen-
     sive-2736099-1.html

20   The IRS recently *clarified* the so-called "market reform restrictions" in
     the ACA. Their interpretation allowed them to fine employers who are
     doing what the president wanted them to do: Offer more employer-sup-
     ported health insurance. See: http://www.marketwatch.com/story/
     what-changes-to-obamacare-could-mean-for-small-business-taxes-
     2015-06-16?mc_cid=289d1b107a&mc_eid=4f671091a3

21   On June 18, 2015, the House of Representatives voted 280-140
     to repeal the Medical Device Tax. The Republican majority was
     joined by 46 Democrats, thus achieving the two thirds major-
     ity necessary to over-rule President Obama's highly vocal veto
     threat. The Senate has resisted considering the repeal. See: http://
     bigstory.ap.org/article/331d8e25dcbd46ffad4336d641c660ae/
     house-ready-repeal-pieces-obama-health-care-law

22   Read Mrs. Kinder's full letter at: http://karrikinder.blogspot.
     com/2014/01/an-update-to-my-open-letter-to-obama.html. It is well
     worth your time.

23   See the publication at: http://illinoisreview.typepad.com/illinoisre-
     view/2013/09/mentally-challenged-24-year-old-denied-care-under-aca.
     html

24   The survey results from the California Medical Association
     can be found at: http://personalliberty.com/2013/12/06/
     report-70-percent-of-california-doctors-wont-participate-in-obamacare

25   Connor Land reported this story in late 2013 at:
     http://mediamatters.org/research/2013/09/27/
     because-fox-asked-here-are-examples-of-people-w/196139

26   Story describes dying cancer patients who were turned
     away from treatment because they had ACA insurance. See:
     http://www.breitbart.com/Big-Government/2014/02/05/
     California-Obamacare-Turning-Cancer-Patients-Away

27   Senator Everett Dirksen, a staunch Republican, was a vocal activist for
     the Civil Rights Acts of 1964 and 1968. He was famous for his offhand
     quip to a reporter, "A billion here, a billion there. Sooner or later, you get
     to some real money."

28   How much proof will satisfy you that I am not exaggerating our danger?
     Try this. "Canada's Supreme Court has ruled that under the "law of the
     land" in Ontario, a government board, not the family or doctors, has
     the ultimate power to pull the plug on a patient." See: "Death Panels
     Alive And Well In Canada And Coming Here," Editorial in Investors'
     Business Daily, 10/22/2013 at: http://news.investors.com/ibd-editori-
     als/102213-676161-death-panels-are-grim-reality-in-canada.htm

29 The article "Cutting costs by killing patients" raised a furor when published on AmericanThinker.com. See: http://www.americanthinker.com/2013/02/cutting_healthcare_costs_by_killing_patients.html. You can also read a recent warning from a British member of the European Parliament titled, "Kill Obamacare, or U.S. healthcare will suffer same fate as Britain," at: http://www.washingtonexaminer.com/kill-ocare-or-it-will-suffer-same-fate-as-nhs/article/2561140

30 The stories of Cantor and Elliot appeared in: http://endoftheamerican-dream.com/archives/10-obamacare-horror-stories-that-are-almost-too-crazy-to-believe

31 When I published the "Seven Reasons" on AmericanThinker.com, there were over seventy irate comments. They were not angry at me, but at the President. See: http://americanthinker.com/2014/08/seven_rea-sons_why_the_aca_pot_keeps_boiling_over.html

32 For details on the four King plaintiffs, see: http://abcnews.go.com/Health/wireStory/sketches-challengers-health-care-law-subsidies-28966707

33 The three dissenting votes in the decision for Burwell were Justices Scalia, Thomas and Alito. For Justice Scalia's quote, see: http://www.newsmax.com/Headline/Scalia-Supreme-Court-SCOTUScare/2015/06/25/id/652159/#ixzz3e7bOMQQg

34 For the official decision, see: King et al *v.* Burwell, Secretary of Health and Human Services, et al, No. 14-114. Argued March 4, 2015. Decided June 25, 2015.

35 Read "TaKing Stock: The Potential Impact of King v. Burwell," by La Couture and Holtz-Eakin at: http://americanactionforum.org/research/taking-stock-the-potential-impact-of-king-v.-burwell

36 In Greek mythology, Panacea was the Goddess of universal remedy, whose touch would heal any ailment. Her father was Asclepius, a human being who was promoted to god status, as the God of Medicine. His snake-entwined staff has become the symbol of a medical healer.

Chapter 10

1 This story is an adaptation of one that circulated on the Internet (original author unknown) and then JD Wolverton commented on the story at: www.dailykos.com/story/2013/04/13/1201511/-willfully-mis-guided-misinformed. His misguided diatribe in fact proved the truth in this analogy, that magical thinking still exists, and how much Kool-aid the author has imbibed.

2   John Harwood wrote in the *New York Times*, November 27, 2011, "Spreading the Wealth; in Democrats' Favor." See: http://thecaucus.blogs.nytimes.com/2011/11/27/spreading-the-wealth-in-democrats-favor.

3   You may have studied Abraham Maslow's "Pyramid" in school. It goes from Physiologic at the base level to Safety, Love/Belonging, then Esteem, and ultimately to Self-actualization. Maslow was a true rebel. (cit. 340) At the insistence of his parents, he enrolled in law school and then immediately dropped out. He defied convention by marrying his first cousin. He plagiarized the concept of self-actualization from his colleague, Kurt Goldstein's 1934 book *The Organism*.

4   For more on thinking systems, including with specific application to healthcare, see citations 543, 548, and 553.

5   Hobbes' famous 1651 tome *Leviathan: The Matter, Forme and Power of a Common Wealth Ecclesiastical and Civil* was one of the building blocks of social contract theory and a major influence on John Locke, whom some call the "Father" of liberalism.

6   I am making a contrast with what the main character and villain, Gordon Gecko played by Michael Douglas, said in the 1987 movie titled *Wall Street*. When taking over, and breaking up, a large corporation, Gecko proclaimed before a shareholders' meeting that, "Greed, in a word, is good!"

7   Samuel Beckett wrote a play titled "Waiting For Godot," about two men talking (there is no action or movement at all) while waiting for a third man to arrive. The third man never shows up. So, *Waiting For Godot* has come to mean waiting for something that never happens. It was hailed as "the most significant English language play of the 20th century" after it premiered in Paris in 1953. Personally, I thought it was boring.

8   Emerson said this during his famous speech titled "The American Scholar," given on request by the Phi Beta Kappa [academic honor] society in Cambridge, Massachusetts on August 31, 1837.

9   Citation #547 shows that only 45% of the in-hospital workforce actually provide (do) care in any form, meaning over half do not. They are "bureaucrats." So there are well over six million bureaucrats physically in hospitals, clinics, etc. Now add the workforces of the FDA, NIH, Medicare, Medicaid, State Legislatures, Congress, and the White House. It is easy to get to more than ten million healthcare bureaucrats.

10   Roberts Higgs discussed the ratchet effect in his 1987 book *Crisis and Leviathan*. [Higgs got the word "Leviathan" —meaning central controlling body—from Hobbes. See note #5 above.] Higgs wrote that most government growth occurred in response to a national crisis, and that the crisis need not be real, only perceived. He went on to say when the

crisis was solved or was shown to be mirage, either way, the government expansion often persisted even then it was no longer 'needed.'

11 Dr. Ben Carson was invited to speak by President Obama at the National Prayer Breakfast. Listen to what he had to say at: http://video. search.yahoo.com/yhs/search?p=Dr.+Ben+Carson%2C+National+Prayer+Breakfast&hspart=FreeCause&hsimp=yhs-shopathome_001.

12 Russ Ackoff was a brilliant contributor to both strategic thinking and management knowledge in the commercial world. His differentiations of data, knowledge, understanding, and wisdom; his four "solves;" his explanation of why analysis is bad for improvement; and more can all be found in citation 4: *Ackoff's Best-His Classic Writings on Management*.

13 Thomas Paine's quote appeared in "The American Crisis, No. 4," published in 1777.

14 I do not like the 1997 dark comedy film *Wag the Dog*, precisely because it seems too close to the truth. The movie tells a story where Presidential sex scandal is about to make headlines. To distract the public, Presidential advisers create a fake war, with Albania. They manipulate the media and the people, plying them with lies, even a war that doesn't exist, all in order to divert their attention away from the President's dalliance. If you haven't seen the film, you probably should.

15 When you read Harwood's "spreading the wealth" (URL is in chapter note #2), you will see that it does not benefit everyone, only the "right people" as defined by the bureaucracy, meaning those who help it grow.

16 And *buying our votes*, to paraphrase Margaret Thatcher, works only until they "run out of others people's money to spend" on purchasing our votes.

Chapter 11

1 Numerous articles are cropping up about concierge medicine, which even has its own web site at: conciergemedicinenews.wordpress.com. Online, check out: http://online.wsj.com/article/SB1000142405270230 3812904577295501951423484.html and http://insurancenewsnet.com/oarticle/2013/06/14/doctors-dump-health-insurance-plans-charge-patients-less-a-384619.html?newswires#.UdGknL-zOix.

2 Leonard, D. Nov. 29, 2012. "Is Concierge Medicine the Future of Health Care?" At: http://www.bloomberg.com/bw/articles/2012-11-29/is-concierge-medicine-the-future-of-health-care#p5

3 You will enjoy reading Von Drehle, D. Dec. 22, 2014. "Medicine Is About to Get Personal," at: http://time.com/topic/solutions-for-america, especially if you are a provider of health care.

4 Dr. Ben Carson's entire speech at: http://yhoo.it/1x0wabI. You probably should watch this video twice. Once to consider what Br. Ben is saying, and a second time to watch the reactions of the President and the First

Lady, both sitting to Carson's right. Also read: http://www.theblaze.com/contributions/dr-ben-carson-is-our-best-choice-for-president.

5   Munro D. Nov. 17, 2014. "U.S. Annual Healthcare Spending Is A Stunning $3.4 Trillion, Says Study." At: http://www.forbes.com/sites/danmunro/2014/11/17/new-deloitte-study-u-s-healthcare-spending-for-2012-was-over-3-4-trillion

6   The 43% was reported by Allison Linn as, "Now it's the 43 percent: Fewer paying no income tax," at: http://www.cnbc.com/id/101015065

7   You probably remember the contemptuous and contemptible Harvard Professor Jonathan Gruber. He was one of the key architects of the ACA. In rare moments of public candor, he exposed his true feelings and actual intent by arrogantly stating, "we just tax insurance companies, they pass on higher prices that offset the tax break they get ... It's a very clever basic exploitation of the lack of economic understanding of the American voter." He even admitted that, "This bill was written in a tortured way to make sure CBO did not score the mandate as taxes." See "Gruber Is Also Wrong On Policy," *Forbes.com*, Nov. 13, 2014 at: http://www.forbes.com/sites/gracemarieturner/2014/11/13/gruber-is-also-wrong-on-policy/?mc_cid=22e7e7fed4&mc_eid=4f671091a3 and http://www.americanthinker.com/articles/2014/11/the_vindication_of_john_roberts.html. His total consulting fee reached well over a million dollars. Thank you, Professor Gruber, for your snake oil.

8   Though you can go directly to hear this snippet of dialogue at https://www.youtube.com/watch?v=4KDSyLT9qKc, I would not recommend it. To get the full flavor, you need first to see the entire episode one, season one, and then view the whole Greater Fool episode. The ninety minutes are well worth your time.

Author's Evidence (References)

1   Ackoff RL, Emery FE. 1972. <u>On Purposeful Systems</u>. Chicago: Aldine-Atherton.

2   Ackoff RL. 1978. <u>The Art of Problem Solving, Accompanied by Ackoff's Fables</u>. Wiley & Sons, New York.

3   Ackoff RL. 1989. From Data to Wisdom. *Journal of Applied Systems Analysis* 16: 3-9.

4   Ackoff RL. 1999. <u>Ackoff's Best-His Classic Writings on Management</u>. Wiley & Sons, New York.

5   Ackoff RL, Rovin S. 2003. <u>Redesigning Society</u>. Stanford Business Books: Stanford, C

6   Aiken LH, Clarke SP, Sloane DM, et al October 23/30, 2002. Hospital Nurse Staffing and Patient Mortality, Nurse Burnout, and Job Dissatisfaction. *Journal of Amer Med Assoc* 286(16): 1987-1993

7   Alexander JA, Fennell M. 1986. Patterns of decision making in multihospital systems. *Jrnl of Health and Social Behavior* 27(1): 14-27.

8   Alexander JA, Lichtenstein R, Oh H, Ullman E. 1998. A causal model of voluntary turnover among nursing personnel in long-term psychiatric settings. *Research in Nursing and Health* 21(5): 415-427.

9   Allen SW, Gauvreau K, Bloom BT, Jenkins KJ. 2003. Evidence-based referral results in significantly reduced mortality after congenital heart surgery. *Pediatrics* 112(1): 24-28.

10 Anderson GF, Hussey PS, Frogner BK, Waters HR. 2005. Health spending in the United States and the rest of the industrialized world. *Health Affairs* 24(4): 903-914.

11 Angell M. 10/13/02. Forgotten domestic crisis. *New York Times*, Op-Ed.

12 Anonymous. Mar/Apr 2003. Research Notes. *Healthcare Exec* 18(2): 42.

13 Anonymous. Jul/Aug 2004. Hospital CEO turnover remains stable in 2003. *Healthcare Executive* 19(4): 65.

14 Argote L, Epple D. 1990. Learning Curves in Manufacturing. *Science* Feb 247: 920–24.

15   Argüellos, JR de P. 2008. "Welfare rights and health care." In: Weisstub DN, Diaz Pintos G. 2008. <u>Autonomy and Human Rights in Health Care</u>. Springer: The Netherlands.

16   Aronson D. 1996-98. Overview of Systems Thinking. www.thinking.net. Accessed Feb 2004.

17   Arndt M, Bigelow B. 2000. The transfer of business practices into hospitals: history and implications. *Advances in Health Care Management* Vol. 1: 339-368.

18   Ashkanasy NM, Broadfoot LE, Falkus S. 2000. Questionnaire measures of organizational culture. In Neal M. Ashkanazy, Celeste P. M. Wilderon, and Mark F. Peterson (Eds.), <u>Handbook of organizational culture and climate</u> (pp. 131-145). Thousand Oaks, CA: Sage Publications

19   Ashmos DP, McDaniel RR. 1991. Physician participation in hospital strategic decision making: The effect of hospital strategy and decision content. *Health Services Research* 26(3): 375-401.

20   Ashmos DP, McDaniel RR. 1996. Understanding the participation of critical task specialists in strategic decision making. *Decision Science* Winter 27(1): 103-121.

21   Ashmos DP, Duchon D, McDaniel RR. 1998. Participation in strategic decision making: The role of organizational predisposition and issue interpretation. *Decision Sciences* 29(1): 25-51.

22   Ashmos DP, Huonker JW, McDaniel RR. 1998. The effect of clinical professional and middle manager participation on hospital performance. *Health Care Management Review* 23(4): 7-20.

23   Ashmos DP, Duchon D, McDaniel RR. 2000. Organizational response to complexity: the effect on organizational performance. *Journal of Organizational Change* 13(6): 577-594.

24   Associated Press, April 4, 2007. "Doctor contrasts his cancer care with uninsured patient who died." Accessed March 2009 at: www.cnn.com/2007/HEALTH/04/04/uninsured.dead.ap/index.html.

25   Associated Press. April 18, 2007. Researchers: Let's Scrap the Internet and Start Over. Accessed May 14, 2007 at: www.foxnews.com/story/0,2933,266124,00.html.

26   Atwater JB, Pittman PH. 2006. Facilitating systemic thinking in business classes. *Decision Sciences Journal of Innovative Education* July, 4(2): 273-292.

27   Axelsson R. 1998. Toward an evidence-based health care management. *International Journal of Health Planning and Management* 13; 307-17

28   Baiker K, Taubman SL, Allen HL, et al. 2013. The Oregon Experiment—Effects of Medicaid on clinical outcomes. *New Engl J Med* 368;18: 1713-22.

29   Baker E. 2001. Learning from the Bristol Inquiry. *Cardiology in the Young* 11: 585-587.

30   Baker T. 1999. <u>Doing Well by Doing Good</u>, Economic Policy Institute, Washington, DC.

31   Baloff, N. 1971. Extension of the Learning Curve—Some Empirical Results. *Operational Research Quarterly* 1971; 22(4): 329–40.

32   Barnard A, Tong K. 2000. The doctor is out. *Boston Globe*, July 9: A18.

33   Barzansky B, Etzel SI. September 5, 2001. Educational programs in the U.S. medical schools 2000-2001. *Journal of American Medical Association* 286(9): 1049-1055

34   Bass CD. 2000. Medicine losing its workhorses. *Albuquerque Journal*, September 17, 2000; page I-2.

35   Barrett R. January 27, 2002. The Apprentices--Construction trades need more people willing to learn while they earn. Albuquerque Journal I-1 & 2.

36   Barron JM, McCafferty S. September 1977. Job search, labor supply, and the quit decision: Theory and evidence. *American Economic Review* 67(4): 683-691.

37   Bartol KM. December 1979. Professionalism as a predictor of organizational commitment, role stress, and turnover: A multidimensional approach. *Academy of Management Journal* 22(4): 815-821.

38   Bates DW, Boyle DL, Vander Vliet MB, et al. 1995. Relationship between medication errors and adverse drug events. *J Gen Int Med* 10(4) 199-205, DOI: 10.1007/BFO2600255.

39   Becker T. 2004. Why pragmatism is not practical. *Journal of Management Inquiry September* 13(3): 224-230. See Jacobs (2004) for companion article.

40   Beedham T. 1996. Why do young doctors leave medicine? *Brit Journal of Hosp Med* 55(11): 699-701. Editorial Comments by Elizabeth Paice 1997; 90(8): 417-418 and by John Davis 1997; 90(10): 585.

41   Begg CB, Cramer LD, Hoskins WJ, Brennan MF. 1998. Impact of Hospital Volume on Operative Mortality for Cancer Surgery. *Journal of the American Medical Association* 280: 1747–51.

42   Beinhocker, ED. 1997. Strategy at the edge of chaos. *The McKinsey Quarterly* Winter #1, pp. 24-40.

43   Beller GA. 2000. Academic Health Centers: The making of a crisis and potential remedies. *J Amer Coll Cardiol* 36:1428-31

44   Bender C, DeVogel S, Blomberg R. 1999. The socialization of newly hired medical staff into a large health system. *Health Care Management Review* 24:95-108.

45   Berenson RA Ginsburg PB, May JH. 2007. Hospital-physician relations: Cooperation, competition, or separation? *Health Affairs* 26(1): w31-w43

46   Berger JE, Boyle RL. November/December 1992. How to avoid the high costs of physician turnover. *MGM Journal* pp. 80-91.

47   Berry LL. 2004. The Collaborative Organization: Leadership lessons from Mayo Clinic. *Organizational Dynamics* 33(3): 228-242.

48   Berta WB, Baker R. 2004. Factors that impact the transfer and retention of best practices for reducing error in hospital. *Health Care Management Review* 29(2): 90-97.

49   (von) Bertalanffy L. 1968. General System theory: Foundation, development, applications. George Braziller, New York, revised edition 1976.

50   Berwick DM. 1989. Continuous Improvement as an ideal in health care. *New England Journal of Medicine* 320(1): 53-56.

51   Berwick DM, Godfrey AB, Roessner J. 1990. Curing Health Care. Jossey-Bass, San Francisco, CA.

52   Bettis RW, Prahahald CK. 1995. The dominant logic: retrospective and extension. *Strategic Management Journal* 16(1): 237-252.

53   Beyer JM, Trice HM: "Using Six Organizational Rites to Change Culture" pages 370-399. In: Kilmann RH, Saxton MJ, Serpa R, et al (1985) Gaining Control of the Corporate Culture. San Franciso: Jossey-Bass.

54   Birkmeyer JD, Finlayson SR, Tosteson AN, et al. 1999. "Effect of Hospital Volume on In-hospital Mortality with Pancreaticoduodenectomy." *Surgery* 125: 250–56

55   Birkmeyer JD, Stukel TA, Siewers AE, et al. 2003. Surgeon volume and operative mortality in the United States. *New England Journal of Medicine* 349: 2117-27.

56   Bisognano M. 2004. What Juran says. One of four essays on "Can the gurus' concepts cure healthcare?" In *Quality Progress* September pp. 33-34.

57   Blackburn R, Rosen B. 1993. Total quality and human resource management: lessons learned from Baldrige award-winning companies. *Academy of Management Executive* 7: 49-66.

58   Blaufuss J, Maynard J, Schollars G. 1992a. Calculating and Updating Nursing Turnover Costs. *Nursing Economic$* January/ February 10(1): 39-45, 78.

59   Blaufuss J, Maynard J, Schollars G. 1992b. Methods of evaluating turnover costs. *Nursing Management* 23(5): 52-59.

60   Bloom J, Alexander JA, Nuchols B. 1992. The effect of the social organization of work on the voluntary turnover rate of hospital nurses in the United States. *Social Science and Medicine* 34(12): 1413-1424.

61   Blumenthal D, Hsiao. September 15, 2005. Privatization and Its Discontents-The Evolving Chinese Health Care System. *The New England Journal of Medicine* 353: 1165-1170.

62   Bole TJ, Bondeson W. 1991. <u>Rights to Health Care</u>. Kluwer Academic Publishers: London.

63   Bolster CJ, Hawthorne G, Schubert P. Nov/Dec 2002. "Executive compensation survey: Can money buy happiness?" *Trustee* 55(10): 8-12.

64   Bonacich, P. 1987. Power and Centrality: A Family of Measures. *American Journal of Sociology* 92(5): 1170-82.

65   Borda RG, Norman IJ. 1997. Factors influencing turnover and absence of nurses: a research review. *International Journal of Nursing Studies* 34(6): 385-394.

66   Bowles S, Gintis H. 1998. The Evolution of Strong Reciprocity. Santa Fe Institute Working Paper, SFI 98-08-073E. Accessed on January 14, 2007 at: http://citeseer.ist.psu.edu/bowles98evolution.html.

67   Bradbury, R. 1966. <u>Farenheit 451</u>. Sundance Books, Littleton, MA. Reprinted 2002.

68   Bragg JE, Andrews IR. 1973. Participative decision-making: An experimental study in a hospital. *Journal of Applied Behavioral Science* 9: 727-735.

69   Brass DJ. 1984. Being in the right place: A structural analysis of individual influence in an organization. *Administrative Science Quarterly*, 29: 518-539.

70   Brass DJ, Burkhardt ME. 1993. Potential power and power use: An investigation of structure and behavior. *Academy of Management Journal* 36(3): 441-470.

71   Brennan TA, Localio AR, Leape LL, et al. 1990. Identification of Adverse Effects Occurring during Hospitalization: A Cross-Sectional Study of Litigation, Quality Assurance, and Medical Records at Two Teaching Hospitals. *Ann Int Med* 112: 221-226.

72   Brennan TA, Sox CM, Burstin HR. 1996. Relation Between Negligent Adverse Events and the Outcomes of Medical-Malpractice Litigation. *N Engl J Med* 335:1963-1967.

73   Brewer LA, Fosburg RG, Mulder GA, Verska JJ (1972) Spinal cord complications following surgery for coarctation of the aorta. *J Thorac Cardiovasc Surg* 64(3): 368-381

74   Brook RH, Lohr KN (1987) Monitoring quality of care in the Medicare Program. *JAMA* 258: 3138-3141.

75   Bristol Royal Infirmary Inquiry Final Report, July 2001; Accessed March 15, 2006 at: www.bristol-inquiry.org.uk/final_report/index. htm.

76   Brockschmidt, FR. 1996. Corporate culture: does it play a role in health care management? *CRNA* 1994; 5:93-6.

77   Broder DS. October 21, 2001. Need for capable government has never been clearer. *Albuquerque Journal,* B2

78   Broder DS. April 17, 2002. Health cost spike can't be ignored. *Albuquerque Journal,* A12.

79   Broder DS. March 18, 2005. Unfunded mandates still plaguing states, cities. *Albuquerque Journal,* #77, A14.

80   Brooks I. 1996. Using rituals to reduce barriers between sub-cultures. *J Mgmt Med* 10(3): 23-30.

81   Brotherton SE, Simon FA, Etzel SI (September 5, 2001) U.S. Graduate medical education 2000-2001. *Journal of American Medical Association* 286(9): 1056-1060.

82   Bruner EM, Ed. 1983. Text, play, and story: the construction and reconstruction of self and society: 1983 Proceedings of the American Ethnological Society. Waveland Press; Prospect Heights, Ill, 1988.

83   Bryan-Brown C, Dracup K. 2001. An Essay on Criticism. *American Journal of Critical Care* 10(1): 1-4

84   Bryson RW, Aderman M, Sampiere JM, Rockmore L, Matsuda T. 1985. Intensive care nurse: Job tension and satisfaction as a function of experience level. *Critical Care Medicine* 13(9): 767-769.

85   Buchan J, Seccombe I. June 13, 1991. The high cost of turnover. *Health Services Journal* 101(5256): 27-28.

86   Buckbinder SB, Wilson M, Melick CF, Powe NR. 2001. Primary care physician job satisfaction and turnover. *American Journal of Managed Care* 7(7): 701-713.

87   Buckingham M, Coffman C. 1999. First, Break All The Rules. Simon and Schuster: New York

88   Burne J. April 16, 2005. Cleaning up MRSA. *The [London] Times,* A12.

89   Burt RS, MJ Miner MJ (eds.) 1983. Applied Network Analysis: A Methodological Introduction. Beverly Hills: Sage.

90   California Healthline, March 20, 2009. "Suit Says Lab Firms Overbilled Medi-Cal for Testing Services." Accessed April 2009 at: http://www.californiahealthline.org/Articles/2009/3/20/Suit-Says-Lab-Firms-Overbilled-MediCal-for-Testing-Services.aspx.

91   Cameron KS, Freeman SJ. 1991. Cultural congruence, Strength, and Type: Relationships to Effectiveness. *Research in Organizational Change and Development* 5: 23-58.

92   Carroll L. Reprinted in 1994. <u>Alice in Wonderland and Through the Looking-Glass.</u> Quality Paperback Book Club: New York.

93   Cassata D. AP, May 8, 2011. Health care costs a hefty price tag for Pentagon. Accessed May 8, 2011 at: http://www.wtop.com/?nid=209&sid=2374508.

94   Carvel J. November 23, 2005. NHS cash crisis bars knee and hip replacements for obese. *Manchester Guardian*, Page 1.

95   Catron D. April 15, 2013. The Wheels Come Off Obamacare. *American Spectator* at: http://spectator.org/archives/2013/04/15/the-wheels-come-off-obamacare.

96   Cavanaugh SJ. 1990. Predictors of Nursing staff turnover. *Journal of Advanced Nursing* 15(3): 373-380.

97   Champy J. 1995. <u>Reengineering Management.</u> HarperBusiness: New York.

98   Charles SC, Gibbons RD, Frisch PR, et al. 1992. Predicting Risk for Medical Malpractice Claims Using Quality-of-Care Characteristics. *Western Journal of Medicine* 157:433-439.

99   Chassin MR. 1998. Is health care ready for six sigma quality? *The Millbank Quarterly* Winter v76 i4 p 565(2)

100   Christenson CM, Bohmer R, Kenagy J. 2000. Will disruptive innovations cure health care? *Harvard Business Review* 78(5): 102-112.

101   Clark RE. 1996. Outcome as a Function of Annual Coronary Artery Bypass Graft Volume. *Annals of Thoracic Surgery* 6(1): 21–26.

102   Claybrook J. 2004. Don't blame lawsuits for rising malpractice insurance rates. *USA Today* Tuesday January 27; p. 19A.

103   Cochrane AL. 1972. <u>Effectiveness and Efficiency: Random Reflections of Health Services.</u> London: Nuffield Trust.

104   Coeling HVE, Wilcox JR. 1988. Understanding organizational culture: A key to management decision-making. *J of Nursing Admin* 18(11): 16-24.

105   Coeling HVE, Simms LM (1993) "Facilitating Innovations at the Nursing Unit Level through Cultural Assessment, Part 1: How to keep Management Ideas from Falling on Deaf Ears." *Journal of Nursing Administration* 23: 46-53.

106   Coeling HVE, Simms LM. 1993. Facilitating Innovation at the unit level through cultural assessment, Part 2. *J of Nursing Admin* 23(5): 13-20.

107   Cohn KH, Peetz ME. 2003. Surgeon frustration: Contemporary problems, practical solutions. *Contemporary Surgery.* 59(2): 76-85.

108   Cohn KH, Gill S, Schwartz R. 2005. Gaining hospital administrators' attention: Ways to improve physician-hospital management dialogue. *Surgery* 137:132-140

109   Cohn KH. 2005. Embracing Complexity, from Cohn KH. *Better Communication for Better Care: Mastering Physician-Administrator Collaboration*, Chicago, Health Administration Press, Pp. 30-38.

110   Coile RC. 1994. "Movement toward managed care leads to shifts in organizational cultures." *Georgia Hospitals Today* 38:4-6.

111   Coleman J, Katz E, Menzel. December 1957. "The diffusion of an innovation among physicians." *Sociometry* 20(4): 253-270.

112   Collins JC, Porras JI. 1997. Built to Last. HarperBusiness: New York.

113   Collins J. 2001. Good to Great. HarperBusiness, New York.

114   Command Paper: CM 5207. July 2001. The Inquiry into the management of care of children receiving complex heart surgery at the Bristol Royal Infirmary—Final Report. Accessed March 2006 at: www.bristol-inquiry.org.uk.

115   Conger JA, Kanungo RN. 1988. The empowerment process: Integrating theory and practice. *Acad of Mgmt Rev* 13: 471-482.

116   Conlin M. Smashing the Clock. YahooBusinessOnLine accessed December 8, 2006 at: http://biz.yahoo.com/special/allbiz120606_article1.html.

117   Connelly LM, Bott M, Hoffart N, Taunton RL. 1997. Methodologic triangulation in a study of nurse retention. *Nursing Research* Sept/Oct 46(5): 299-302

118   Conner D. 1990. Corporate culture: Healthcare's change master. *Healthcare Executive* 5: 28-9.

119   Consumer Reports February 2007. "Get better care from your doctor." Accessed January 4, 2006 at: www.ConsumerReports

120   Cooke R, Szumal J. 1991. Measuring normative beliefs and shared behavioral expectations in organizations: The Reliability and Validity of the Organizational Culture Inventory. *Psychological Reports* 72: 1299-1330.

121   Cooke RA, Szumal J. 2000. Using the organizational culture inventory to understand operating cultures of organizations. In Neal M. Ashkanasy, Celeste P. M. Wilderon, and Mark F. Peterson (Eds.), Handbook of organizational culture and climate (pp. 147-162). Thousand Oaks, CA: Sage Publications.

122   Cotton JL, Vollrath DA, Froggatt KL, Lengnick-Hall ML, Jennings KR. 1988. Employee participation: Diverse forms and different outcomes. *Academy of Management Review*, 13(1): 8-22.

123   Coulson JD, Seddon MR, Readdy WF. March 2008. Advancing Safety in pediatric cardiology—Approaches Developed in Aviation. *Congenital Cardiology Today*, Vol 6, No. 3, Pp 1-10.

124   Coutu DL. 2002. The anxiety of Learning. [Interview with Edgar Schein]. *Harvard Business Review* March, pp 100-106.

125   Covey, SR 1989. The Seven Habits Of Highly Effective People. Simon & Schuster: New York.

126   Cox, A. 1987. The Court and the Constitution. Houghton Miflin: Boston.

127   Cuny J (2005) "Failure to Rescue—2004 Benchmarking Project." Accessed June 2005 at: www.uhc.edu.

128   D'Aunno T, Alexander JA, Laughlin C. 1996. Business as usual? Changes in Health Care's workforce and organization of work. *Hospital and Health Services Administration* 16: 3-18.

129   Dalton DR, Todor WD. 1979. Turnover turned over: An expanded and positive perspective. Acade*my of Management Review* 4: 225-35.

130   Damasio AR. 1994. Descartes' Error: Emotion, Reason and the Human Brain. Avon Books: New York.

131   Danzon PM. 1985. *Medical Malpractice: Theory, Evidence and Public Policy*. Harvard University Press, Cambridge, MA.

132   Danzon PM. 1986. New evidence on the frequency and severity of medical malpractice claims. Rand Corporation, Santa Monica, CA. R-3410-ICJ.

133   Daschle, T Greenberger, SS, Lambrew JM. 2008. Critical: What We Can Do About the Health-Care Crisis. New York: St. Martin's Press.

134   Davidson M. 1983. Uncommon Sense—The Life and Thought of Ludwig von Bertalanffy (1901-1972), Father of General Systems Theory. Tarcher, Inc., Los Angeles.

135   Dauten D. 2001. The cost of being ordinary. Dale@dauten.com

136   Davies HTO, Nutley SM, Mannion R. 2000. Organizational Culture and Quality of Health Care. *Quality in Health Care* 9: 111-9.

137   Davis TRV: "Managing Culture at the Bottom" pages 163-182. In: Kilmann RH, Saxton MJ, Serpa R, et al (1985) Gaining Control of the Corporate Culture. San Franciso: Jossey-Bass.

138   Davis SM: "Culture Is Not Just and Internal Affair" pages 137-147. In: Kilmann RH, Saxton MJ, Serpa R, et al (1985) Gaining Control of the Corporate Culture. San Franciso: Jossey-Bass.

139   Deal TE, Kennedy AA. 1982. Corporate Culture: Rites and Rituals of Corporate Life. Perseus Publishing, Cambridge, MA.

140   Deal TE: "Cultural Change: Opportunity, Silent Killer, or Metamorphosis?" pages 292-331. In: Kilmann RH, Saxton MJ, Serpa R, et al (1985) Gaining Control of the Corporate Culture. San Franciso: Jossey-Bass.

141   Deal TE, Kennedy AA. 1999. The New Corporate Cultures. Perseus Books, Reading MA.

142   Deems RS. 1999. Calculating true cost of employee turnover. *Balance* 3(3): 13

143   Degeling P, Kennedy J, Hill, M. 1998. Do Professional Subcultures Set the Limits of Hospital Reform? *Clinician in Management* 7: 89-98.

144   Denison DR, Spreitzer GM. 1991. Organizational culture and organizational development: a competing values approach, *Research in Organizational Change and Development,* 5:1-21.

145   Desjardins RE. 1997. Does your corporate culture contribute to the problem? *Food & Drug Law Journal* 52:169-71.

146   Dilts DM, Sandler AB. 2006. The "Invisible" Barriers to Clinical Trials: The impact of Structural, Infrastructural, and Procedural Barriers to Opening Oncology Clinical Trials," *Journal Clinical Oncology,* 24(28): 4545-52.

147   Dixon K. 2004. "HMOs bringing back unpopular cost controls-Survey." Reuters, 8/10/04. Accessed 8/10/04 at: http://news.yahoo.com/news? tmpl=story&cid=571&u= /nm/20040811/hl_nm/health_hmos_study.

148   Dobyns L. March 20, 2006. "How hospitals heal themselves." Accessed 9/16/06 at: www.managementwisdom.com/goodnews.html.

149   Donabedian A. 1985. Explorations in Quality Monitoring and Assessment and Monitoring—Volume III, The Methods and Findings of Quality Assessment and Monitoring: An Illustrated Analysis. Health administration Press, Ann Arbor, MI.

150   Douglas CH, Higgins A, Dabbs, C, Walbank M. 2004. Health impact assessment for the sustainable futures of Salford. *J Epidemiol Community Health* 58: 642-648.

151   Dowd S, Davidhizar R. 1997. Change management—organizational culture as change factor. *Administrative Radiology Journal* 16:20-5.

152   Drake D, Fitzgerald S, Jaffe M. 1993. Hard Choices—Health Care at What Cost? Andrews & McMeel: Kansas City.

153   Droste TM. 1996. Merging corporate cultures in integrated systems. *Medical Network Strategy Report* 5:1-3.

154   Dwore, RB Dwore RB, Murray BP. 1989. Turnover at the top: Utah hospital CEOs in a turbulent era. *Hosp Health Serv Admin* Fall, 34(3): 333-351.

155   Dyer, Jr. WG: The Cycle of Cultural Evolution in Organizations, pages 200-229. In: Kilmann RH, Saxton MJ, Serpa R, et al (1985) Gaining Control of the Corporate Culture. San Franciso: Jossey-Bass.

156   Dyer, WG. 1987. Team building: Issues and alternatives (2nd ed.). Reading, MA: Addison Wesley Publishing Company.

157   Ebon M. 1987. The Soviet Propaganda Machine. McGraw-Hill: New York.

158   Edmondson AC. 1996. "Learning from mistakes is easier said that done: Group and organizational influences on the detection and correction of human error." Journal of Appl Behav Sci 32(1): 5-28.

159   Edmondson, AC. 2008. "The Competitive Imperative of Learning." Harvard Business Review July-August: 60-67.

160   Edmonton TV. Opposition demand health care review. Accessed 3/11/11: http://calgary.ctv.ca/servlet/an/local/CTVNews/20110311/CGY_health_care_110311/20110311/?hub=CalgaryHome.

161   Ellis SG, Weintraub W, Holmes D, Shaw R, Block PC, King SB. 1997. Relation of Operator Volume and Experience to Procedural Outcome of Percutaneous Coronary Revascularization at Hospitals With High Interventional Volumes. Circulation 95: 2479–84.

162   Engstrom P. 1995. Cultural differences can fray the knot after MDs, hospitals exchange vows. Medical Network Strategy Report 4:1-5.

163   Epstein RA. 1999. Mortal Peril—Our Inalienable Right To Health Care? Perseus Books: Cambridge, MA.

164   Eubanks P. 1991. Identifying your hospital's corporate culture. Hospitals 65: 46.

165   European Observatory on Health Care Systems 2000. Health Care Systems in Transition: Belgium. Copenhagen: World Health Organization. Accessed on February 10, 2006 at: http://www.euro.who.int/document/e71203.pdf.

166   Evans M. October 18, 2004. For a limited time only. Modern Healthcare. 34 (42): 6-8.

167   Feldstein PJ. 2005. Health Care Economics, 6th ed. Thomson Delmar Learning. Clifton, NY. Pp. 207-208.

168   Fennell ML, Alexander J. September 1987. "Organization boundary spanning and institutionalized environments." Academy of Management Journal 30: 456-476.

169   Ferlie E, Fitzgerald L, Wood M. 2000. Getting evidence into clinical practice: an organizational behavior perspective. Journal of Health Services Research & Policy 5(2): 96-102.

170   Ferlie EB, Shortell SM. 2001. Improving the quality of health care in the United Kingdom and the United States: A framework for change. Millbank Quarterly 79(2): 281-315.

171   Ferrara-Love R. 1997. Changing organizational culture to implement organizational change. *Journal of Perianesthesia Nursing* 12: 12-6.

172   Fickeisen DH. Winter 1991. Learning How to Learn, An Interview with Kathy Greenberg. The Learning Revolution (IC#27) by the Context Institute. Page 42. www.context.org/ICLIB/IC27/Greenbrg. htm. Accessed December 2004.

173   Fiol CM, O'Connor EJ, Aguinis. 2001. All for one and one for all? The development and transfer of power across organizational levels. *Academy of Management Review*, 26(2): 224-242.

174   Fitzgerald FS. 1936. The Crack-Up. New Directions Books: New York. Reprinted 1945.

175   Flowers VS, Hughes CL. July/August 1973. Why employees stay. *Harvard Business Review* pp. 49-60.

176   Fletcher B, Jones F. 1992. Measuring Organizational Culture: The Cultural Audit. *Managerial Auditing Journal* 7 (6): 30-6.

177   Forrester JW. 1971. The counterintuitive behavior of social systems. *Technology Review* 73(3): 52-68.

178   Franczyk A. 2000. Turnover in hospital CEOs brings change to healthcare industry. *Business First*. Buffalo: Jul24, 2000. Vol 12, Iss. 44, pp1-2.

179   Freiberg K, Freiberg J. 1996. Nuts! Southwest Airlines' Crazy Recipe for Business and Personal Success. Broadway Books: New York.

180   Friedman EA, Adashi EY. December 15, 2010. The right to health as the unheralded narrative of health care reform. *JAMA* 304(23): 2639-2640.

181   Galloro V. February 19, 2001. Staffing outlook grim-High turnover expected to continue in skilled nursing, assisted living. *Modern Healthcare* 31(8): 64.

182   Garside P. 1998. Organizational context for quality: Lesson from the fields of organizational development and change management. *Quality in Health Care* 7(Suppl): S8-15

183   Garson A. 2001. The Edgar Mannheim Lecture: From white teeth to heart transplants: evolution in international concepts of the quality of healthcare. *Cardiology in the Young* 11: 601-608.

184   Gawande A. 12/30/07. A Lifesaving checklist. NewYorkTimes. com at: http://www.nytimes.com/2007/12/30/opinion/30gawande. html?_r=2&oref=slogin.

185   Gawande A. January 24, 2011. Can we lower medical costs by giving the neediest patients better care? *New Yorker Online*. Accessed March 7, 2011 at: http://www.newyorker.com/ reporting/2011/01/24/110124fa_fact_gawande?currentPage=all.

186   Gawande A. May 26, 2011. Cowboys and Pit Crews. The New Yorker. Accessed at: http://www.newyorker.com/online/blogs/newsdesk/2011/05/atul-gawande-harvard-medical-school-commencement-address.html.

187   Gentry WD, Parkes KR. 1982. Psychologic stress in the ICU and non-intensive unit nursing: A review of the past decade. *Heart & Lung* 11(1): 43-47.

188   George JM, Jones GR. 1996. The experience and work and turnover intentions: Interactive effects of value attainment, job satisfaction, and positive mood. *Journal of Applied Psychology* 81(3): 318-325.

189   Gerowitz M, Lemieux-Charles L, Heginbothan C, ans Johnson B. 1996. Top Management Culture and Performance in Canadian, UK and U.S. Hospitals. *Health Services Management Research* 6 (3): 69-78.

190   Glaser S, Zamanou S, Hacker K. 1987. Measuring and Interpreting Organizational Culture. *Management communication quarterly* 1 (2): 173-98.

191   Glazner L. 1992. Understanding corporate cultures: use of systems theory and situational analysis. *AAOHN Journal* 40:383-7.

192   Goldman RL. 1992. The reliability of peer assessment of quality of care. *JAMA* 267(7): 958-960.

193   Goldman DP, McGlynn EA. 2005. U.S. Health Care: Facts about Cost, Access and Quality. Rand Report CP484.1. Accessed December 29, 2006 at: www.rand.org/pubs/corporate-pubs/CP484.1.

194   Goldratt E, Cox J (1984). The Goal-A Process of Ongoing Improvement. North River Press, Great Barrington, MA.

195   Goldsmith J. 2003. Digital Medicine: Implications for Healthcare Leaders. Chicago: Health Administration Press.

196   Goldworth A. 2008. "Human rights and the right to health care." In: Weisstub DN, Diaz Pintos G. 2008. Autonomy and Human Rights in Health Care. Springer: The Netherlands.

197   Goodman EA, Boss RW. 1999. Burnout dimensions and voluntary and involuntary turnover in a health care setting. *Journal of Health & Human Services Administration* Spring, 21(4): 462-471.

198   Goodman J. November 8, 2010. "Being stupid about prices." Accessed May 2011 at: http://healthblog.ncpa.org/stupid-about-prices.

199   Goodman JM, Jones GR. 1996. The experience and work and turnover intentions: Interactive effects of value attainment, job satisfaction, and positive mood. *Journal of Applied Psychology* 81(3): 318-325.

200   Goold M, Campbell A. 2002. Do you have a well-designed organization?" *Harvard Business Review* March 117-124.

201   Gordon GG: "The Relationship of Corporate Culture to Industry Sector and Corporate Performance" pages 103-125. In: Kilmann RH, Saxton MJ, Serpa R, et al (1985) <u>Gaining Control of the Corporate Culture</u>. San Franciso: Jossey-Bass.

202   Gray AM, Phillips VL, Normand C. 1996. The costs of nursing turnover: Evidence from the British National Health Service. *Health Policy* 38: 117-128

203   Greco PJ, Eisenberg JM. 1993. Changing Physicians' Practices. *New England Journal of Medicine* 329(17): 1271-1274

204   Greene J. February 6, 1995. Clinical integration increases profitability, efficiency—study. Modern Healthcare, page 39

205   Griffeth RW, Hom PW, Hall TE. 1981. "How to estimate employee turnover costs. Personnel 58(4): 43-52.

206   Griffeth RW, Hom PW. 2001. <u>Retaining Valued Employees</u>. Sage Publications, Thousand Oaks, CA.

207   Groupman J. 2007. <u>How Doctors Think</u>. Houghton Miflin: New York.

208   Grout JR. 2003. Preventing medical errors by designing benign failures. *Joint Commission Journal on Quality and Safety* 29(7): 354-362.

209   Gustafson BM. 2001. Improving staff satisfaction ensures PFS success. *Healthcare Financial Management* 55(7): 66-68.

210   Hadley J, Mitchell JM, Sulmasy DP, Bloch MG. 1999. Perceived financial incentives, HMO market penetration, and physicians' practice styles and satisfaction. *Health Services Research* Vol. 34, #1, Part II: 307-321.

211   Haft H. "The right to Basic Health Care is Afforded to Every Citizen of the United States." *Physician Executive* Jan-Feb 2003. http://find-articles.com/p/articles/mi_m0843/is_1_29/ai_96500897.

212   Hale C. May 7, 2003. NHS Chiefs 'forced into trickery.' *London Times*, P 6.

213   Hall ET, Hall MR. 1990. <u>Understanding Cultural Differences</u>. Intercultural Press, Yarmouth, Maine.

214   Hammer M, Champy J. 1994. <u>Reengineering the Corporation-A Manifesto for Business Revolution</u>. HarperBusiness, New York, NY.

215   Hammer M. 2001. <u>The Agenda</u>. Crown Business, New York.

216   Hannan, EL, Racz M, Kavey R-E, et al. 1998. Pediatric Cardiac Surgery: The Effect of Hospital and Surgeon Volume on In-hospital Mortality. *Pediatrics* 101(6): 963-69.

217   Hariri S, Prestipino AL, Rubash HE. April 2007. The Hospital-Physician Relationship: Past, Present and Future. *Clinical Orthopaedics and Related Research* 457: 78-86.

218   Harrison, R. 1972. Understanding Your Organization's Character. *Harvard Business Review* 5 (3): 119-28.

219   Hart LG, Robertson DG, Lishner DM, Rosenblatt RA. 1993. CEO turnover in rural northwest hospitals. *Hosp Health Serv Admin* Fall; 38(3): 353-374.

220   Hatch AP. 2005. CBS abandons Murrow Ideals. *Albuquerque Journal* October 20; Page A13.

221   Hawkes, Nigel. January 18, 2002. Patients get power to select surgeons. *London Times*

222   Heinlein R. 1963. Glory Road. Avon Books: New York. Page 253

223   Heinlein, R.1966. The Moon Is A Harsh Mistress. Berkley Publishing Corp: New York.

224   Henninger D. January 10, 2003. "Marcus Welby doesn't live here anymore." *Wall Street Journal*, Page A10.

225   Herzberg F. 1968. One more time: How do you motivate employees? *Harvard Business Review* Reprint RO301F in *Best of HBR* January 2003 pp. 3-11.

226   Herzlinger RE. 1997. Market-Driven Health Care. Addison-Wesley Publ., Reading MA.

227   Herzlinger RE. November 26, 2003. Back in the USS.R. *Wall Street Journal*, Opinion, Vol 240, A16.

228   Heskett JL, Sasser WE, Schlesinger LA: The Service Profit Chain, Free Press, NY, 1997.

229   Hill LD, Madara JL. November 2, 2005. Role of the Urban Academic Medical Center in U.S. Health Care. *JAMA* 294(17): 2219-2220.

230   Hilts PJ. June 23, 1993. Health-care Chiefs' pay rises at issue." *New York Times*, pg D2.

231   Hoban CJ. 2002. From the lab to the clinic: Integration of pharmacogenics into clinical development. *Pharmacogenics* 3(4): 429-436. .

232   Hock D. 1999. Birth of the Chaordic Age. Berrett-Koehler: San Francisco.

233   Hofstede G, Neuijen B, Ohayv DD, Sanders G. 1990. Measuring organizational cultures: A qualitative and quantitative study across twenty cases." *Administrative Science Quarterly* 35:286-316.

234   Howard PK. July 31, 2002. There is no 'right to sue'. *Wall Street Journal*, Page 13.

235   Hughes L. 1990. Assessing organizational culture: Strategies for external consultant. *Nursing Forum* 25 (1): 15-19.

236   Hume SK. 1990. Strengthening the corporate culture. *Health Progress* 71:15-6, 19.

237   Huselid MA, Jackson SE, Schuler RS. 1997. Technical and strategic human resource management effectiveness as determinants of firm performance. *Academy of Management Journal* 40(1): 171-188.

238   Hutchinson J, Runge W, Mulvey M,et al. 2004. *Burkholderia cepacia* infections associated with intrinsically contaminated ultrasound gel: The role of microbial degradation of parabens. *Infect Contr and Hosp Epidem* 25: 291-296

239   Iglehart J. 1998. Forum on the future of academic medicine: Session III—Getting from Here to There. *Academic Medicine* 73 (2): 146-151

240   Ingersoll GL, Kirsch JC, Merk SE, et al. 2000. Relationship of Organizational culture and Readiness for Change to Employee Commitment to the Organization. *Journal of Nursing Admin* 30 (1); 11-20.

241   Irvine DM, Evans MG. 1995. Job satisfaction and Turnover among nurses: Integrating research findings across studies. *Nursing Research* July/August 44(4): 246-253.

242   Jacobs DC. 2004. A pragmatist approach to integrity in business ethics. *Journal of Management Inquiry September* 13(3): 215-223.

243   Jain KK. 2005. Personalised medicine for cancer: from drug development into clinical practice. *Expert Opin. Pharmacother.* 6(9): 1463-1476.

244   Janssen PPM, de Jonge J, Bakker AB. 1999. Specific determinants of intrinsic work motivation, burnout and turnover intentions: a study among nurses. *Journal of Advanced Nursing* 29(6): 1360-1369.

245   Jenkins KJ, Gauvreau K, Newburger JW, et al. 2002. Consensus-based method for risk adjustment for surgery for congenital heart disease. *Journal of Thoracic & Cardiovascular Surgery* January 123: 110-118.

246   Jha AK, Perlin JB, Kizer KW, Dudley RA. May 29, 2003. Effect of the transformation of the Veterans Affairs Health Care System and the quality of care. *New England Journal of Medicine* 348(2): 2218-2227.

247   Jiang HJ, Friedman B, Begun JW. 2006. Factors Associated with High-Quality/Low-Cost Hospital Performance. *Journal of Health Care Finance* Spring: 39-51

248   Johnson DE. 1997. Medical group cultures pose big challenges. *Health Care Strategic Management* 15:2-3.

249   Johnson J, Billingsley M. 1997. Reengineering the corporate culture of hospitals." *Nursing & Health Care Perspectives* 18:316-21.

250   Johnson L. 1999. Cutting costs by managing turnover. *Balance, The Journal of the American College of Health Care Administrators.* Sept/Oct 1999 pp 21-23.

251   Johnson, Rep. Nancy. Febr 2001. Congressional Outlook: Nursing Shortages. *Hospital Outlook* 4(2): 7.

252   Johnson S. 2001. Emergence. New York: Simon & Schuster, 2001.

253   Joiner KA, Wormsley S. March 2005. Strategies for Defining Financial Benchmarks for the Research Mission in Academic Health Centers. *Academic Medicine* 80(3): 211-217.

254   Joiner KA. March 2005. A Strategy for allocating central funds to support new faculty recruitment. *Academic Medicine* 80(3): 218-224.

255   Joiner KA. July 2004. Sponsored-Research Funding by Newly Recruited Assistant Professors: Can It Be Modeled as a Sequential Series of Uncertain Events? *Academic Medicine* 79(7): 633-643.

256   Joiner KA. July 2004. Using Utility Theory to Optimize a Salary Incentive Plan for Grant-Funded Faculty, *Academic Medicine* 79(7): 652-660.

257   Jollis JG, Peterson ED, DeLong ER, et al. 1994. The Relation Between the Volume of Coronary Angioplasty Procedures at Hospitals Treating Medicare Beneficiaries and Short-Term Mortality. *NEJM* 331: 1625–29.

258   Jones WT. 1961. The Romantic Syndrome: Toward a new method in cultural anthropology and the history of ideas. The Hague: Martinus Wijhaff.

259   Jones CB. 1990a. Staff nurse turnover costs: Part I, a conceptual model. *Journal of Nursing Administration,* 20(4): 18-22. AND

260   Jones CB. 1990b. Staff nurse turnover costs: Part II, measurement and results. *Journal of Nursing Administration,* 20(5): 27-32.

261   Jones CB. 1992. Calculating and Updating Nursing Turnover Costs." *Nursing Economic$* January/February 10(1): 39-45, 78.

262   Jones KR, DeBaca V, Yarbrough M. 1997. Organizational culture assessment before and after implementing patient-focused care. *Nursing Economics* 1997; 15:73-80.

263   Jones WJ. 2000. The 'Business'—or 'Public Service'—of Healthcare. *J Healthcare Mgmt* 45(5): 290-293.

264   Jorgensen A: "Creating changes in the corporate culture: case study." *AAOHN Journal* 1991; 39:319-21.

265   Jung CG. 1973. Four archetypes: Mother/Rebirth/Spirit/Trickster. Princeton University Press: Princeton, NJ.

266   Jurkiewicz CL, Knouse SB, Giacalone RA (March/April 2001) "When an employee leaves: The effectiveness of clinician exit inter-views and surveys." *Clinical Leadership Mgmt Review* 15(2): 81-84.

267   Kaiser Family Foundation, March 2009. Health Care Costs—A Primer. Accessed March 2009 at: www.kff.org.

268   Kan JS, White RI, Mitchell SE, Gardner TJ. 1982. Percutaneous balloon valvuloplasty: a new method for treating congenital pulmonary valve stenosis. *New Engl J Med* 307: 540-542.

269   Kallestad B. Fall 2006. *Leadership Quarterly*, Associated Press Report accessed January 1, 2007 at: http://news.yahoo.com/s/ap/bad_bosses

270   Karcz A, Korn R, Burke MC, et al. (1996) Malpractice Claims Against Emergency Physicians in Massachusetts: 1975-1993. *Am J Emergency Medicine* 14: 341-345.

271   Kauffman, Draper. 1980. Systems One: An Introduction to Systems Thinking. SA Carlton, Minneapolis, MN.

272   Kauffman SA. 1995. At Home in the Universe. Oxford University Press, NY.

273   Keeler EB, Brook RH, Goldberg GA, Kamberg CJ, Newhouse JP (1985) "How free care reduced hypertension in the Health Insurance Experiment." *JAMA* Oct. 11, 1985; Vol. 254: 1926-1931.

274   Keeton WP, Dobbs DB, Keeton RE, Owen DG. 1984. *Prosser and Keeton on The Law of Torts.* Fifth Edition. West Publishing Co., St. Paul, MN.

275   Kellerman B. 2007. What every leader needs to know about followers. *Harvard Business Review* December, pp. 84-91.

276   Kerr S. 1975. On the folly of rewarding A While hoping for B. *Academy of Mgmt Journal* 18: 769-783.

277   Kesner KA, Calkin JD. 1986. Critical care nurses' intent to stay in their positions. *Research in Nursing & Health* 9: 3-10.

278   Kessler DP, McClellan MB. 2002. How liability law affects medical productivity. *J Med Economics* 21(6): 931-955.

279   Kiel JM. 1998. Using data to reduce employee turnover. *Health Care Supervisor* 16(4): 12-19.

280   Kilmann RH, Saxton MJ, Serpa R, et al. 1985. Gaining Control of the Corporate Culture. San Franciso: Jossey-Bass. See: Kilmann RH: "Five Steps of Closing Culture Gaps" pages 351-369 and Kilmann RH, Saxton MJ and Serpa R: "Conclusion: Why Culture Is Not Just a Fad" pages 421-432.

281   Kinard J, Little B. 1999. Are hospitals facing a critical shortage of skilled workers? *Health Care Supervisor* 17(4): 54-62.

282   King L. 1963. The Growth of Medical Thought. University of Chicago Press: Chicago.

283   Kissick WL. 1995. Medicine and Management. Bridging the cultural gaps. *Physician Executive* 21:3-6.

284   Kite M. June 03, 2003. Fat people will have to diet if they want to
        see the doctor. *London Times.*

285   Klaasen P. March 14, 2007. Accessed at: www.cnn.com/2007/
        HEALTH/04/04/uninsured.dead.ap/index.htm.

286   Klein LW, Schaer GL, Calvin JE, et al. 1997. Does Low Individual
        Operator Coronary Interventional Procedural Volume Correlate
        with Worse Institutional Procedural Outcome? *Journal of the
        American College of Cardiology* 30, no. 4: 870–77.

287   Klienke JD. 1998. Bleeding Edge-The Business of Health Care in the
        New Century. Aspen Publishers, Gaithersburg, MD

288   Klienke JD. September/October 2005. Dot-Gov: Market failure and
        the creation of a national health information technology system.
        Health Affairs 24(5): 1246-1262.

289   Klingle RS, Burgoon M, Afifi W, Callister M. 1995. Rethinking
        how to measure organizational culture in the hospital setting.
        The Hospital Culture Scale. *Evaluation & the Health Professions*
        18:166-86.

290   Kosmoski KA, Calkin JD. 1986. Critical care nurses' intent to stay
        in their positions. *Research in Nursing & Health* 9: 3-10.

291   Kotter JP, Schlesinger LA. 1979. Choosing strategies for change."
        *Harvard Business Review Mar-*Apr 57(2): 106-114

292   Kotter JP, Heskett JL. 1992. Corporate Culture and Performance.
        Free Press: New York.

293   Kouzes JM, Posner BZ. 1997. The Leadership Challenge; Jossey-
        Bass Inc., San Francisco

294   Krackhardt D, Porter LW. 1985. When friends leave: A structural
        analysis of the relationship between turnover and stayers' attitudes.
        Administrative Science Quarterly, 30, 42-61.

295   Kraman SS, Hamm G. 1999. Risk management: Extreme honesty
        may be the best policy. *Ann Int Med* 131(12): 963-967.

296   Kravitz RL, Rolph JE, Petersen L. 1997. Omission-Related
        Malpractice Claims and the Limits of Defensive Medicine. *Medical
        Care Res & Review* 54: 456-471.

297   Krauthammer C. 1998. Driving the best doctors away. *Washington
        Post* January 9; p A21.

298   Kübler-Ross, E. 1969. On Death and Dying. Touchstone: New York.

299   Lacour-Gayet F, Clarke D, Jacobs J, et al. 2004. The Aristotle Score:
        a complexity-adjusted method to evaluate surgical results. *European
        Journal of Cardio-Thoracic Surgery* 25: 911-924.

300   Landis SE. January 3, 2006. Do the Poor deserve life support?
        Accessed December12, 2006 at www.slate.com/toolbar.aspx?action.

301   Landon BE, Reschovsky J, Blumenthal D. 2003. Changes in career satisfaction among primary care and specialist physicians, 1997-2001. *JAMA* 289(4): 442-449.

302   Landro, Laura. December 22, 2003. Six prescriptions for what's ailing U.S. Health care. *Wall Street Journal* Vol 242 #122, pp. A1 & A10.

303   Langer E. 1997. The Power of Mindful Learning. Perseus Books: New York.

304   Langwell KM, Werner JL. 1984. Regional Variations in the Determinants of Professional Liability Claims. *Journal of Health Politics, Policy and Law* 9:475-88.

305   LaPar DJ, Bhamidipati C, Mery CM et al. 2010. Primary Payer Status Affects Mortality For Major Surgical Operations. American Surgical Association meeting. Accessed May 2013 at: http://www.americansurgical.info/abstracts/2010/18.cgi.

306   Laurance J. December 6, 2004. NHS Revolution: nurses to train as surgeons. *The Independent* (London)

307   Lawry TC. May 1995. Making culture a forethought. *Health Progress* 76(4): 22-25, 48

308   Lazlo E. 1972. The Systems View of the World. G Braziller: New York.

309   Leape LL. December 21, 1994. Error in Medicine. *JAMA* 272(3): 1851-1857.

310   Lee RT, Ashforth BE. 1996. A meta-analytic examination of the correlates of the three dimensions of job burnout. *Journal of Applied Psychology* 81: 123-133.

311   Lerner J. 1997. *The Rush Initiative for Mediation of Medical Malpractice Claims.* 11 CBA Record 40.

312   Levering R, Moskovitz M. 1993. *The 100 Best Companies to Work for in America*; Doubleday, New York.

313   Levinson W, Roter DL, Mullooly JP, et al. 1997. Physician-Patient Communication: The Relationship with Malpractice Claims Among Primary Care Physicians and Surgeons. *JAMA* 277: 553-559.

314   Levitt S, Dubner S. 2005. Freakonomics—A Rogue Economist Explores the Hidden Side of Everything. Harper Collins: New York.

315   Lewin K. 1947. Frontiers in group dynamics. *Human Relations*, Volume 1, pp. 5-41

316   Linn A. February 12, 2005. Biggest Airbus Jet is Too Big. *Albuquerque Journal*, No. 43, C-1. 4

317   Lisney B, Allen C. 1993. Taking a snapshot of cultural change. *Personnel Management* 25 (2): 38-41.

318   Litwinenko A, Cooper CL: "The impact of trust status on corporate culture." *Journal of Management in Medicine* 1994; 8:8-17.

319   Localio AR, Lawthers AG, Brennan TA, et al. 1991. Relation
        between malpractice claims and adverse events due to negligence:
        Results of the Harvard Medical Practice Study III. *N Engl J Med*
        325: 245-251.

320   Loop FD. 2001. On medical management. *J Thorac Cardiovasc Surg*
        121(4): S25-S28.

321   Lorsch JW: "Strategic Myopia: Culture as an Invisible Barrier to
        Change" pages 84-102. In: Kilmann RH, Saxton MJ, Serpa R, et al
        (1985) Gaining Control of the Corporate Culture. San Franciso:
        Jossey-Bass.

322   Louis MR: "Sourcing Workplace Cultures: Why, When, and How"
        pages 126-136-102. In: Kilmann RH, Saxton MJ, Serpa R, et al
        (1985) Gaining Control of the Corporate Culture. San Franciso:
        Jossey-Bass.

323   Luft HS, Bunker, Enthoven AC. 1979. Should operations be
        regionalized? The empirical relation between surgical volume and
        mortality. *N Engl J Med* Dec 20; 301(25): 1364-69.

324   Luft, HS. 2003. From observing the relationship between volume
        and outcome to making policy recommendations—Comments on
        Sheikh. *Medical Care* 41(10): 1118-1122.

325   Lurie N, Manning WG, Peterson C, Goldberg GA, Phelps CA,
        Lilliard L. 1987. Preventive Care: Do we practice what we preach?
        American Journal of Public Health 77:801-804.

326   Maarse H, Paulus A. Has solidarity survived? A comparative analy-
        sis of the effect of social health insurance reform in four European
        countries. *J Health, Politics, Policy and Law* 2003; 28(4): 585-614.

327   Machiavelli N. 1513. The Prince. Wordsworth Editions,
        Hertfordshire, England, 1993.

328   Mackenzie S. 1995. "Surveying the organizational culture in a NHS
        trust." *J Mgmt Med* 9(6): 69-77.

329   Mackey J. August 11, 2009. "The Whole Foods Alternative to
        Obamacare." Wall Street Journal Online. http://online.wsj.com/
        article/SB10001424052970204251404574342170072865070.html.

330   Maclean, N. 1992. Young Men and Fire. University of Chicago:
        Chicago. Mahony L, Sleeper LA, Anderson PAW, et al. 2006.
        Pediatric Heart Network: A primer for the conduct of multicenter
        studies in children with congenital & acquired heart disease.
        Pediatric Cardiology 27: 191-198.

331   Malcolm L, Wright L, Barnett, Hendry C. 2003. Building a success-
        ful partnership between management and clinical leadership: expe-
        rience from New Zealand. *British Medical Journal* 326: 653-654.
        Downloaded 31 August 2006 from doi:10.1136/bmj.326.7390.653.

332   Manger LN 2005. <u>A History of Medicine</u>. Taylor & Francis: New York.

333   Mann EE, Jefferson KJ. "Retaining staff: Using turnover indices and surveys. *JONA* 1988; 18(7,8): 17-23.

334   Mano-Negrin R (2001) "An occupational preference model of turnover behavior: The case of Israel's medical sector employees." *Journal of Management in Medicine* 15(2): 106-114.

335   Marmot M. 2004. <u>The Status Syndrome—How Social Standing Affects Our Health and Longevity</u>. Holt & Co.: New York.

336   Marsh R Mannari H. 1977. Organizational commitment and turnover: A predictive study. *Administrative Science Quarterly* 22: 57-75.

337   Martin, N. June 4, 2007. "Smokers who won't quit denied surgery" by Nicole Martin in the *Daily Telegraph Today*, June 4, 2007, at: http://www.telegraph.co.uk/global/ main.jhtml?xml=/global/2007/06/04/nhealth04.xml.

338   Martin TE. 1979. A contextual model of employee turnover intentions. *Academy of Management Journal* 22(2): 313-324.

339   Martin HJ: "Managing Specialized Corporate Cultures" pages 148-162. In: Kilmann RH, Saxton MJ, Serpa R, et al (1985) <u>Gaining Control of the Corporate Culture</u>. San Franciso: Jossey-Bass.

340   Maslow AH. 1943. A theory of human motivation. *Psychological Rev* 50: 370-396.

341   Matthews, M. June 2, 2011. Irrational exuberance and accountable care organizations. Accessed 6/3/11 at: http://blogs.forbes.com/merrill matthews/2011/06/02/irrational-exuberance-and-accountable-care-organizations.

342   Matus JC, Frazer GH. 1996. Job satisfaction among selected hospital CEOs." *The Health Care Supervisor* September 15(1): 41-60.

343   May L. 1993. Institutions and the transformation of personal values. Are the traditional values of caring and service in jeopardy? *Clinical Laboratory Management Review* 7:191-3.

344   Matus JC, Frazer GH. 1996. Job satisfaction among selected hospital CEOs. *The Health Care Supervisor* September 15(1): 41-60.

345   McCallum KL. May 7, 2001. All the good doctors always leave. *Medical Economics* 78(9): 55-6, 58, 61

346   McConnell CR. 1999. Staff turnover: Occasional friend, frequent foe, and continuing frustration. *Health Care Manager* 18(1): 1-13.

347   McDaniel RR. 1997. Strategic Leadership: A View from quantum and chaos theories. *Health Care Management Review* 22(1) 21-37.

348   McDaniel RR, Driebe DJ. 2001. Complexity Science and Health Care Management. *Advances in Health Care Management* 2: 11-36.

349   McFadden KL, Towell ER, Stock GN. 2004. Critical success factors for controlling and managing Hospital Errors. *Quality Management Journal* 2004; 11(1) 61-73.

350   McGinn R. May 10, 2006. Malpractice Caps Limit Care. *Albuquerque Journal*, #130, Page A11.

351   McGrath PD, Wennberg DE, Malenka DJ, et al. 1998. Operator Volume And Outcome in 12,998 Percutaneous Coronary Interventions. *Journal of American College of Cardiology* 31(3): 570–76.

352   McIntyre N, Popper KB. 1989. The critical attitude in medicine: the need for a new ethics. *British Medical Journal* 287:1919-1923

353   McMurray, AJ. 2003. The relationship between organizational climate and organizational culture. *Journal of the American Academy of Business*, 3: 1-8.

354   Melcher AJ (1976) Participation: A critical review of research findings. *Human Resource Management* Summer: 12-21.

355   Melville A. 1980. Job satisfaction in general practice: Implications for prescribing. *Social Sciences & Medicine* 14A(6): 495-499

356   Merry M. 1998. Will you manage your organization's culture, or will it manage you? *Integrated Healthcare Report* pp. 1-11.

357   Merry MD. 2004. What Deming Says. One of four essays on Can the gurus' concepts cure healthcare? In *Quality Progress* September pp. 28-30.

358   Meschievitz CS. 1994. Efficacious or Precarious? Comments on the Processing and Resolution of Medical Malpractice Claims in the United States, 3 Annals Health L. 123, 127-130.

359   Messinger DS, Bauer CR, Das A, et al. 2004. The maternal lifestyle study: Cognitive, motor, and behavioral outcomes of cocaine-exposed and opiate-exposed infants through three years of age. *Pediatrics* 113: 1677-168.

360   Metzloff TB. 1992. *Alternate Dispute Resolution Strategies in Medical Malpractice.* 9 Alaska L. Rev. 429, 431.

361   Metzloff TB. 1996. *The Unrealized Potential of Malpractice Arbitration,* 31 Wake Forest L. Rev. 203, 204, 1996.

362   Metzloff TB. 1997. *Empirical Perspectives on Mediation and Malpractice.* 60-WTR Law & Contemp. Probs. 107, 110-113. *See also,* N.C. Gen. Stat. § 7A-38.1 (1998).

363   Millenson ML. 1999. <u>Demanding Medical Excellence: Doctors and accountability in the Information Age</u>. University of Chicago Press.

364   Millenson, ML. 2003. The Silence. *Health Affairs* 22(2): 103-112.

365   Miller, J 1995. <u>Lockheed Martin's Skunk Works</u>. Midland Publishers: Leicester, England.

366   Miller RH, Lipton HL, Duke KS, Luft HS. 1996. Update Special Report, The San Diego Health Care System: A Snapshot Of Change. *Health Affairs* 15.1: 224-229.

367   Miller MM. December 25, 2003. Don't look for responsible leadership under tree. *Albuquerque Journal* Vol 358, A12.

368   Miller WL, Crabtree BF, McDaniel R, et al. May 1998. Understanding change in primary care practice using complexity theory. *Journal of Family Practice* 46(5): 369-376.

369   Mingardi A. November 17, 2006. A drug price path to avoid. *Albuquerque Journal*, A13.

370   Mintzberg H. 1983. <u>Structuring of Organizations</u>. Englewood Cliff: Prentice Hall.

371   Mirvis PH Lawler EE. 1977. Measuring the financial impact of employee attitudes. *Journal of Applied Psychology* 62:1-18.

372   Mitroff II and Kilmann RH: "Corporate Taboos and the Key to Unlocking Culture" pages 184-199. In: Kilmann RH, Saxton MJ, Serpa R, et al (1985) <u>Gaining Control of the Corporate Culture</u>. San Franciso: Jossey-Bass.

373   Mobley WH, Horner SO, Hollingsworth AT. 1978. Evaluation of precursors of hospital employee turnover. *Journal of Applied Psychology* 63(4): 408-414.

374   Mobley WH. 1982. <u>Employee Turnover: Causes, Consequences and Control</u>. Addison-Wesley, Reading, MA.

375   Moffit RE. Dec 23, 2010. "Doctors, Patients, and the New Medicare Provisions." Heritage Foundation lectures #1174 (September 23, 2010): 1-8. Accessed January 2011 at: http://report.heritage.org/h1174.

376   Moore WW. 1991. Corporate culture: modern day rites & rituals." *Healthcare Trends & Transition* 2:8-10, 12-3, 32-3.

377   Morrissey, E. November 15, 2012. What free market medicine looks like. Accessed December 2012 at: http://hotair.com/archives/2012/11/15/video-what-free-market-medicine-looks-like.

378   Mosca L, Appel LJ, Benjamin EJ et al. 2004. Evidence-based guidelines for cardiovascular disease prevention in women. American Heart Association scientific statement. *Arterioscler Thromb Vasc Biol* Mar; 24(3): 29-50.

379   Mott DA. 2000. Pharmacist job turnover, length of service, and reasons for leaving, 1983-1997. *Amer Journal of Health-System Pharmacy* 57(10): 975-984.

380   Mowday RT, Steers RM, Porter LW. 1979. The measurement of organizational commitment. *Journal of Vocational Behavior* 14: 224-27.

381   Mowday RT. 1981. Viewing turnover from the perspective of those who remain: The relationship of job attitudes to attributions of the causes of turnover. *Journal of Applied Psychology* 66(1): 120-123.

382   Mullainathan S, Thaler RH. "Behavioral Economics." Accessed November 2006 at: http://introduction.behaviouralfinance.net/MuTh.pdf.

383   Mullaney, TJ. October 31, 2005. This Man Wants to Heal Health Care. *Business Weekly* 3957, p 74.

384   *Murphy v Board of Med. Examiners*, 949 P.2d 530 (Ariz. Ct. App. 1997).

385   Naisbitt J. 1982. Megatrends. Warner Books: New York.

386   Neilsen DM. 2004. What Crosby says. One of four essays on Can the gurus' concepts cure healthcare? In *Quality Progress* September pp. 26-27

387   Nelson, Dave. October 2005. Baldrige—Just What The Doctor Ordered. *Quality Progress*, pp 69-75.

388   Neuhauser PC. 1999. Strategies for changing your corporate culture." [Re: *Front of Hlth Serv Mgmt* Fall; 16(1): 3-29] *Front of Hlth Serv Mgmt* 16:33-7.

389   Neumann E. 1955. The Great Mother: An analysis of archetype. Princeton, NJ: Princeton University Press.

390   NICE Manuals: Guide to the Methods of the Technology Appraisal. Accessed March 16, 2007 at: www.nice.org.uk.

391   Ocasio W, Kim H. 1999. The circulation of corporate control: Selection of functional backgrounds of new CEOs in large U.S. manufacturing firms. *Administrative Science Quarterly* 44(3): 532-563.

392   O'Connell C. 1999. A culture of change or a change of culture? *Nursing Administration Quarterly* 23:65-8.

393   O'Connor JP, Nash DB, Buehler ML, Bard M. 2002. Satisfaction higher for physician executives who treat patients, survey says. *The Physician Executive* May-June pp. 16-21

394   O'Daniell EE. 1999. Energizing corporate culture and creating competitive advantage: a new look at workforce programs. *Benefits Quarterly* 15:18-25.

395   Ogbrun PL, Julian TM, Brooker DC, et al. 1988. Perinatal Medical Negligence Closed Claims from the St. Paul Company, 1980-1982. *Journal of Reproductive Medicine* 33: 608-611.

396   O'leary, DS. 1988. Will a New Federal Climate Affect Joint Commission Confidentially Policy? *Joint Commission Perspectives* Septembre/Octobre 8. 9-10: 2-4.

397   Oliva R. 2002. Tradeoffs in response to work pressure in the service industry. *IEEE Engineering Management Review* First Quarter pp.53-62.

398   Oliver WW. Kicking The Malpractice Tort Out of Court. *Wall Street Journal*, March 19, 2013. Available at: http://online.wsj.com/article/ SB10001424127887323869604578366770324716616.html.

399   Orentlicher D. 2000. Medical Malpractice: Treating the Causes Instead of the Symptoms. *Medical Care* 38: 247-249.

400   *Orlando Sentinel*, April 26, 1998. "Doctor's Victory Revives Proponents of Quality Care, p. A-21.

401   *Orlando Gen. Hospital v Department of Health and Rehabilitative Servs.*, 567 So. 2d 962, 965 (Fla Dist. Ct. Appl. 1990).

402   Osnos E. September 28, 2005. In China, health care is scalpers, lines, debt. *Chicago Tribune*, Section 1, pp 1 & 6.

403   Owen H. Winter 1991. Learning as Transformation. The Learning Revolution (IC#27) by the Context Institute. Page 42. www.context. org/ICLIB/IC27/Owen.htm. Accessed December 2004.

404   Pascale RT, Sternin J. 2005. Your Company's Secret Change Agents. *Harvard Business Rev.* 83(5): 73-81.

405   Pathman DE, Williams ES, Konrad TR. 1996. Rural physician satisfaction: its sources and relation to retention." *Journal of Rural Health* 12(5): 366-377.

406   Pathman DE, Konrad TR, Williams ES, et al. 2002. Physician job satisfaction, dissatisfaction, and turnover. *Journal of Family Practice* 51:593.

407   Patterson KJ and Wilkins AL: "You Can't Get There From Here: What Will Make Culture-Change Projects Fail" pages 262-291. In: Kilmann RH, Saxton MJ, Serpa R, et al (1985) Gaining Control of the Corporate Culture. San Franciso: Jossey-Bass.

408   Payne, J. April 9, 2007. Poor Getting Brushoff for Care. *Albuq Journal*, P. C1.

409   Pearson SD, Rawlins, MD. November 23/30, 2005. Quality, Innovation, and Value for Money: NICE and the British National Health Service. *JAMA* 294(20): 2618-2622.

410   Peirce JC. 2000. The paradox of physicians and administrators in health care organizations. *Health Care Management Review* 2(1): 7-28

411   Peters TJ, Waterman RH. 1982. In Search of Excellence. Warner Books, New York, NY.

412   Petrock F. 1990. Corporate culture enhances profits." *HR Magazine* 35:64-6.

413   Pettigrew A. 1979. "On Studying Organizational Culture." *Administration Science Quarterly* 24:570-81.

414   Pettigrew A, Ferlie E, McKee L. 1992. Shaping Strategic Change-Making change in large organizations. The Case of the National Health Service. Sage Publ., London

415   Pfeffer J. April 1976. Beyond management and the worker: The Institutional Function of Management. *Academy of Management Review* 1(2): 36-46

416   Pfeffer J. 1994. Competitive Advantage Through People. Harvard Business School Press: Boston.

417   Pfeffer J, Sutton RI. 2000. The Knowing-Doing Gap. Harvard Business School Press, Boston, MA.

418   Phibbs CS, Bronstein JM, Buxton E, Phibbs RH. 1996. The Effects of Patient Volume and Level of Care at the Hospital of Birth on Neonatal Mortality. *Journal of the American Medical Association* 276: 1054–59.

419   Phillips RI. 1974. The informal organization in your hospital. *Radiologic Technology* 46(2): 101-106

420   Phillips K. August 16, 2005. Hospitals increasing tapping female executives. Nursezone.com. At: http://nursezone.com/include/PrintArticle.asp?articleid=12529.

421   Pies R. March 13. 2100. Health Care is a Basic Human Right--Almost Everywhere but Here. Accessed March 14, 2011 at: http://www.opednews.com/articles/Health-Care-is-a-Basic-Hum-by-Ronald-Pies-110313-363.html.

422   Porter LW, Steers RM, Mowday RT. 1974. Organizational commitment, job satisfaction, and turnover among psychiatric technicians. *Journal of Applied Psychology* 59(5): 603-609.

423   Porter ME, Teisberg EO. 2006. Redefining Health Care—Creating Value-Based Competition on Results. Harvard Business School Publishing, Boston, MA.

424   Posner KL, Caplan RA, Cheney FW. 1996. Variation in Expert Opinion in Medical Malpractice Review. *Anesthesiology* 85: 1049-1054.

425   Potetz L, Cubanski J, Neumen. February 2011. Medicare Spending and Financing, Kaiser Family Foundation.

426   Prescott PA. 1986. Vacancy, stability, and turnover of registered nurses in hospitals. *Research in Nursing & Health* 9: 51-60.

427   Price JL, Mueller CW. 1981. A causal model of turnover for nurses. *Acad of Mgmt Journal* 24(3): 543-565.

428   Pritchard RD, Campbell KM, Campbell DJ. 1977. Effects of extrinsic financial rewards on intrinsic motivation. *Journal of Applied Psychology* 62(1): 9-15.

429   Proenca EJ. 1996. Market orientation and organizational culture in hospitals." *Journal of Hospital Marketing* 11:3-18.

430   Prosser WP, Dobbs DB, Keeton RE, Owen DG. 1984. Prosser and Keeton on The Law of Torts, Fifth Edition, West Publishing Cp: St Paul, MN.

431   Provan KG. July 1984. Interorganizational cooperation and decision making autonomy in a consortium multi-hospital system. *Academy of Management Review* 9(3): 494-504.

432   Putkowski D. 2009. Universal Coverage. Hawser Press: Media, PA.

433   Quam L, Dingwall R, Fenn P. 1987. Medicine and the Law, Medical Malpractice in Perspective: I—The American Experience. *British Medical Journal* 294: 1529-1532.

434   Quigley W. December 17, 2001. London Report: Medical missteps compound in child's death. *Albuquerque Journal*, p A2

435   Quigley W. October 28, 2002. The health of health care. Quoting Martin Hickey, former Lovelace CEO. *Albuquerque Journal*, Outlook, pp. 3, 9

436   Quinn RE, Spreitzer GM. 1991. The Psychometrics of the competing values culture instrument and an analysis of the impact of organizational culture on quality of life. *Research in Organizational Change and Development*, 5:115-142.

437   Rabinowitz S, Hall DT. 1977. Organizational research on job involvement. *Psych Bull* 84:265-288.

438   Rand A. 1957. Atlas Shrugged. Signet books: New York.

439   Rasmussen, Tom. 29 July 2005. A Mandated Burden." *The Wall Street Journal* A-13.

440   Reinhardt UE. May 18, 2011. Would privatizing Medicare lead to better cost controls? *New York Times Online* accessed at: http://economix.blogs.nytimes.com/author/uwe-e-reinhardt.

441   Reno R. 2001. Health-care system is beyond repair. *Albuquerque Journal*, August 20. A8.

442   Report to Congress: Improving Incentives in the Medicare Program, June 2009. Medicare Payment Advisory Commission, Washington, DC.

443   Rentsch JR. 1990. Climate and culture: Interactions and qualitative differences in organizational meanings." *Journal of Applied Psychology*, 75, 668-681.

444   Richards BC, Thomasson G. 1992. Closed Liability Claims Analysis and the Medical Record. *Obstetrics & Gynecology* 80: 313-316.

445   Rickles D, Hawe P, Shiell A. 2007. A Simple guide to chaos and complexity. *J Epidemiol. Community Health* 61: 933-937, accessed November 20 2007 at: doi:10.1136/jech.2006.054254.

446   Riter RN. 1994. Changing organizational culture." *Journal of Long-term Care Administration* 22:11-13.

447   Roberts G. 11/23/05. "Overweight patients to be denied NHS hip operations." *London Times*, Page 2.

448   Robinson s. 1981. Off the Wall at Callahan's. Tor Books, NY. Page 36.

449   Rogers EM. 1983. Diffusion of Innovation. The Free Press, New York.

450   Rosch E, Lloyd BB [eds.] (1978) Cognition and Categorization. Hillsdale, N.J.: Lawrence Erlbaum.

451   Rothermel RC. May 1993. "Mann Gulch Fire: A Race That Couldn't Be Won." Accessed March 2006 at: http://www.fs.fed.us/rm/pubs/int_gtr299.

452   Rousseau L. 1984. What are the real costs of employee turnover? *CA Magazine* (Toronto) 117(2): 48-55.

453   Rowley TJ. 1997. Moving beyond dyadic ties: A network theory of stakeholder influences. *Academy of Management Review.* 22: 887-910.

454   Rucci AJ, Kirn SP, Quinn RT. 1998. The employee-customer-profit chain at Sears. *Harvard Business Review* Jan/Feb, 83-97.

455   Sackett DL, Rosenberg WM, Gray JA, Haynes RB, Richardson WS. 1996. Evidence based medicine: what it is and what it isn't. *British Medical Journal* 312(7023): 71-2.

456   Sales, AL, Mirvis PH. 1984. When cultures collide: Issues in acquisition, in Managing Organizational Transitions by JR Kennedy, Publ: RD Irwin, Homewood, IL. pp. 107-133.

457   Sapienza AM: "Believing Is Seeing: How Culture Influences the Decisions Top Managers Make" pages 66-83. In: Kilmann RH, Saxton MJ, Serpa R, et al (1985) Gaining Control of the Corporate Culture. San Franciso: Jossey-Bass.

458   Sathe V: "How to Decipher and Change Corporate Culture" pages 230-261. In: Kilmann RH, Saxton MJ, Serpa R, et al (1985) Gaining Control of the Corporate Culture. San Franciso: Jossey-Bass.

459   Schein EH: "How culture forms, develops and changes," pages 17-43. In: Kilmann RH, Saxton MJ, Serpa R, et al (1985) Gaining Control of the Corporate Culture. San Franciso: Jossey-Bass.

460   Schelling TC. 1960. The Strategy of Conflict. Cambridge: Harvard University Press.

461   Schneider J. 1976. The "greener grass" phenomenon: Differential effects of a work context alternative on organizational participation and withdrawal intentions. *Organizational Behavior and Human Performance* 16: 308-33.

462   Schwartz WB, Komesar NK. 1978. Doctors, Damages and Deterrence. *New Engl J Med* 298: 1282-1289.

463   Schyve PM. 2004. What Feigenbaum says. One of four essays on
        "Can the gurus' concepts cure healthcare?" In *Quality Progress*
        September pp. 30-33.
464   Scott RA, Aiken LH, Mechanic D, Moravcsik J. 1995.
        Organizational aspects of caring. *Millbank Quarterly* 73(1): 77-95
465   Scott T, Mannion R, Davies H, Marshall M. 2003. The Quantitative
        Measurement of Organizational Culture in Health Care: A Review
        of the Available Instruments. *Health Services Research* 38(3):
        923-38.
466   Seago J. 1997. Organizational Culture in Hospitals: Issues in
        Measurement. *Journal of Nursing Measurement* 5 (2): 165-78.
467   Senge PM. 1990. The Fifth Discipline-The Art and Practice of the
        Learning Organization. Currency Doubleday, New York.
468   Sfikas PM. 1998. Are Insurers Making Treatment Decisions? *JADA*
        129: 1036-1039.
469   Shader K, Broome ME, Broome CD, et al. April 2001. Factors
        influencing satisfaction and anticipated turnover for nurses at an
        academic medical center. *Journal of Nursing Administration* 31(4):
        210-216.
470   Shanahan MM. 1993. A comparative analysis of recruitment and
        retention of health care professionals. *Health Care Management
        Review* 18(3): 41-51.
471   Shanks H (1968) *The Art and Craft of Judging—The Decision of
        Learned Hand.* Macmillan Co., New York.
472   Shannon v. McNulty, M.D., 718 A.2d 828, (S.Ct.Pa. 1998) and
        Corporate Health Insurance, Inc. v. Texas Department of Insurance,
        215 F.3d 526 (5th Cir.2000) (rehearing den'd, 2000 WL 1035524)
        and Tex Civ. Prac. & Rem., § 88.001 et seq.; Tex. Ins. Code, art.
        20A.09(e), 20A.12(a & b); 20A.12A, 28. 58A § 6(b & c), 28.58A §
        6A, 21.58A § 8(f), 21.58C.
473   Shaw GB. 1913. *Preface to* The Doctor's Dilemma, Penguin:
        Baltimore. Reprinted in 1954.
474   Sheikh A, Hurwitz B. 1999. A national database of medical errors.
        Journal of the Royal Society of Medicine November 92: 554-555.
475   Sheikh, K. 2003. Reliability of provider volume and outcome
        associations for healthcare policy. *Medical Care* October, 41(10):
        1111-1117.
476   Sherer JL. 1994. Corporate cultures. Turning 'us versus them' into
        'we.'" *Hospitals & Health Networks* 68:20-2, 24, 26-7.
477   Shortell SM. Fall 1988. The evolution of hospital systems:
        Unfulfilled promises and self-fulfilling prophecies. *Medical Care
        Review* 45: 745-772

478   Shortell SM, Gillies RR, Anderson DA, Mitchell JB, Morgan KL. Winter 1993. Creating organized delivery systems: The barriers and facilitators. *Hospital & Health Services Administration* 38(4): 447-466

479   Shortell SM, O'Brien JL, Carman JM, et al. June 1995. Assessing the impact of continuous quality improvement/total quality management: Concept versus implementation. *Health Services Research* 30(2): 377-401.

480   Shortell S. March 1997. Commentary on: "Physician-Hospital integration and the economic theory of the firm" by JC Robinson. *Medical Care Research and Review* 54:3-24.

481   Shortell SM, Bennett CL, Byck GR. 1998. Assessing the impact of continuous quality improvement on clinical practice: What it will take to accelerate progress. *Millbank Quarterly* 76(4): 593-624.

482   Shortell S, Waters T, Budetti P, Clarke K. 1998. Physicians as double agents: Maintaining trust in an era of multiple accountabilities. *JAMA* 23: 1102-1108.

483   Shortell SM, Gillies RR, Anderson DA, Morgan-Erickson K, Mitchell J. 2000. Remaking Health Care in America: The Evolution of Organized Delivery Systems. San Francisco: Jossey-Bass.

484   Shortell SM, Jones RH, Rademaker AW, et al. 2000. Assessing the Impact of Total Quality management and Organizational Culture on Multiple Outcomes of Care for Coronary Artery Bypass Graft Surgery Patients. *Medical Care* 38 (2): 207-17.

485   Shortell SM, Zazzali JL, Burns LR, et al. 2001. "Implementing Evidence-Based Medicine: The Role of Market Pressures, Compensation Incentives, and Culture in Physician Organization. *Medical Care* 39 (7, Supplement): I-62-78.

486   Shorter E. 1985. Bedside Manners. Simon & Schuster: New York

487   Sieveking N, Bellet W, Marston RC. 1993. Employees' view of their work experience in private hospitals. *Health Services Mgmt Research* 6 (2): 129-38.

488   Simone JV. 1999. Understanding Academic Medical Centers: Simone's Maxims. *Clinical Cancer Research* 5:2281-2285

489   Simunovic M, To T, Theriault, M, et al. Pediatric Cardiac Surgery: The Effect of Hospital and Surgeon Volume on In-hospital Mortality. *Pediatrics* 1998; 101(6): 963-69.

490   Simons R, Davila A. 1998. "How high is your return on management? *Harvard Business Review* 76; 70-80

491   Smircich, L. 1985. Is the concept of culture a paradigm for understanding organizations and ourselves? In P. J. Frost, L. F. Moore, M. R. Louis, C. C. Lundberg, and J. Martin (Eds.), Organizational Culture (pp. 55-72). Beverly Hills, Calif.: Sage.

492   Smith B, West K. 2002. Death certification: an audit of practice
        entering the 21st century. *Journal of Clinical Pathology* 55: 275-279.

493   Smith GCS, Pell JP. 2003. Parachute use to prevent death and major
        trauma related to gravitational challenge: systematic review of
        randomized controlled trials. *British Medical Journal* 327: 1459-61.

494   Smith GP. 2008. "Accessing health care resources: Economic,
        Medical, Ethical and Socio-legal challenges." In: Weisstub DN, Diaz
        Pintos G. <u>Autonomy and Human Rights in Health Care</u>. Springer:
        The Netherlands.

495   Smith FJ. 1977. Work attitudes as predictors of attendance on a
        specific day. *Journal of Applied Psychology* 62(1): 16-19.

496   Smith HL, Yourstone S, Lorber D, Mann B. 2001. Managed care
        and medical practice guidelines: The thorny problem of attaining
        physician compliance. In <u>Advances in Health Care Management</u>,
        Vol II, Elsevier Science Ltd., New York, NY

497   Smith HL, Waldman JD, Fottler M, Hood JN. 2005. Strategic
        Management of Internal Customers: Building Value through
        Human Capital and Culture." *Journal of Nursing Administration*
        November, **In Press**

498   Soffel D, Luft HS. 1993. Anatomy of health care reform proposals.
        Western Jrnl of Medicine 159: 494-500.

499   Spear S, Bowen HK. 1999. Decoding the DNA of the Toyota
        Production system. *Harvard Business Review* September/October
        pp. 97-106.

500   Spear SJ. September 2005. Fixing Healthcare from the Inside,
        Today. *Harvard Business Review*, pp. 2-16.

501   Steel RP, Ovalle NK. 1984. A Review and meta-analysis of research
        on the relationship between behavioral intentions and employee
        turnover. *Journal of Applied Psychology* 69(4): 673-686.

502   Steiger B. Nov/Dec 2006. Survey Results: Doctors Say Morale Is
        Hurting. *Physician Executive*. Pp. 6-15. Accessed January 23, 2006
        at: www.acpe.org/education/surveys/morale/morale.htm.

503   Sterman JD. 2002. Systems dynamics modeling: Tools for learning
        in a complex world. *IEEE Engineering Management Review* First
        Quarter pp. 42-52.

504   Sterman J. 2006. Learning from evidence on a complex world. *Amer
        Journal of Public Health* 96: 505-514.

505   Stevenson, K. 2000. Are your Practices Resistant to Changing Their
        Clinical Culture? *Primary Care Report* 2 (5): 19-20.

506   Stocking B. 1992. Promoting change in clinical care. *Quality in
        health care* 1: 56-60.

507   Stoller JK, Orens DK, Kester L. March 2001. The impact of turn-over among respiratory care practitioners in a health care system: Frequency and associated costs. *Respiratory Care* 46(3): 238-242.

508   Stossel T, Shaywitz D. July 9, 2006. Biotech Bucks Don't Corrupt Researchers. Reprinted from the *Washington Post* in the *Albuquerque Journal*, Page B3.

509   Stowe JD. 2000. Staff turnover or staff retention: Understanding the dynamics of generations at work in the 21st century. *Canadian Veterinary Journal* 41(10): 803-808

510   Stross, C. 2004. The Family Trade. Tom Doherty Associates Books: New York.

511   Stubblefield A. 2005. The Baptist Healthcare Journey to Excellence, Wiley & Sons: Hoboken, NJ.

512   Studdert DM, Thomas EJ, Burstin HR, Orav J, Brennan TA. 2000. Negligent Care and Malpractice Claiming Behavior in Utah and Colorado. *Medical Care* 38: 250-260.

513   Studer, Q. 2003. Hardwiring Excellence. Gulf Breeze, FL. Fire Starter Publishing

514   Surowiecki J. 2004. The Wisdom of Crowds. Anchor Books: New York.

515   Swift B, West K. 2002. Death certification: an audit of practice entering the 21st century. *Journal of Clinical Pathology* 55: 275-279

516   Tai TWC, Bame SI, Robinson CD. 1998. Review of nursing turn-over research, 1977-1996. *Soc. Sci. Med.* 47(12): 1905-1924.

517   *Tallahassee Mem'l Reg'l Med. Ctr. v. Cook*, 109 F.3d 693 (11th Cir. 1997).

518   Taragin MI, Wilczek AP, Karns ME, Trout R, Carson JL. 1992. Physician demographics and the risk of medical malpractice. *Amer J Med* 93: 537-542.

519   Taragin MI, Sonnenberg FA, Karns ME, Trout R, Shapiro S, Carson JL. 1994. Does Physician Performance Explain Interspecialty Differences in Malpractice Claim Rates? *Medical Care* 32: 661-667.

520   Tate, NJ. 2012. Obamacare Survival Guide. Humanix Books: West Palm Beach, FL.

521   Thomas C, Ward M, Chorba C, Kumiega A (1990) "Measuring and interpreting organizational culture." *Journal of Nursing Administration* 20(6): 17-24.

522   Thomas EJ, Studdert DM, Burstin HR, et al. 2000. Incidence and Types of Adverse Events and Negligent Care in Utah and Colorado. *Medical Care* 38: 261-271.

523   Thompson, Clive. December 10, 2006. Bicycle Helmets Put You At Risk. *The New York Times Magazine*, Section 6, Page 36.

524   Tribus M. 1992. The germ theory of management. *National Institute for Engineering Management & Systems,* Publication #1459

525   Tribus M. February 1992. Reducing Deming's 14 Points to practice. *Quality First.* National Institute for Engineering Management and Systems, NSPE Publication #1459

526   Trice HM, Beyer JM (1984) "Studying organizational cultures through rites and ceremonials." *Academy of Management Review* 9(4): 653-669.

527   Trigg B. February 25, 2011. "Make Health Care A Right for All." *Albuquerque Journal,* A9.

528   Tucker R, McCoy W, Evans. 1990. Can questionnaires Objectively Assess Organizational Culture? *Journal of Managerial Psychology* 5 (4): 4-11.

529   Tuchman B. 1984. The March of Folly. Alfred Knopf: New York.

530   US General Accounting Office (GAO). Impact on Hospital and Physician Costs Extends Beyond Insurance. *Medical Liability* 95.169 (1995): 01-17.

531   Uttal B (October 17, 1983) "The Corporate Culture Vultures." *Fortune* pp. 66-72.

532   Van der Merwe R, Miller S. 1971. The Measurement of Labour Turnover. *Human Relations* 24(3): 233-253

533   Van Watson GH. 2002. Peter F. Drucker: Delivering Value to Customers. *Quality Progress* May pp. 55-61.

534   Vergara GH. 1999. Finding a compatible corporate culture. *Healthcare Executive* 14:46-7.

535   Vitkine B. 2012. Inside the dramatic collapse of Greece's healthcare system. Accessed December 2012 at: http://www.businessinsider.com/collapse-of-greeces-healthcare-system-2012-12.

536   Waldman JD, Young TS, Pappelbaum SJ, Turner SW, Kirkpatrick SE, George L. 1982. Pediatric cardiac catheterization with 'same-day' discharge. *Amer J Cardiol* 50:800-804.

537   Waldman JD, Pappelbaum SJ, George L, et al. 1984. Cost-containment strategies in congenital heart disease. *West J Med* 141:123-126.

538   Waldman JD, Ratzan RM, Pappelbaum SJ. 1998. Physicians must abandon the *illusion* of autonomy.... *Pediatric Cardiology* 19:9-17.

539   Waldman JD. 2001. Aim with Echo in Pulmonary Atresia (The echo machine *works* in the cath lab.) *Pediatric Cardiology* 22(2): 91-92.

540   Waldman JD, McCullough G. 2002. A Calculus of *Unnecessary* Echocardiograms—Application of management principles to healthcare. *Pediatric Cardiology* 23: 186-191.

541   Waldman JD, Spector RA. 2003. Malpractice claims analysis yields widely applicable principles. *Pediatric Cardiology* 24(2): 109-117.

542   Waldman JD, Smith HL, Hood JN. 2003. Corporate Culture —The missing piece of the healthcare puzzle. *Hospital Topics* 81(1): 5-14.

543   Waldman JD, Schargel F. 2003. Twins in Trouble: The need for system-wide reform of both Healthcare and Education. *Total Quality Management & Business Excellence* October, 14(8): 895-901.

544   Waldman JD, Yourstone SA, Smith HL. 2003. Learning Curves in Healthcare. *Health Care Management Review* 28(1): 43-56.

545   Waldman,JD, Smith HL, Kelly F, Arora S. 2004. The Shocking Cost of Turnover in Healthcare. *Health Care Management Review* 29(1): 2-7.

546   Waldman JD, Arora S. 2004. Retention rather than turnover—A Better and Complementary HR Method. *Human Resource Planning* 27(3): 6-9.

547   Waldman JD, Hood JN, Smith HL, et al. 2004. Changing the Approach to Workforce Movements: Application of Net Retention Rate. *Journal of Applied Business and Economics.* 24(2): 38-60.

548   Waldman JD, Schargel F. 2006. Twins in Trouble (II): Systems Thinking in Healthcare and Education. *Total Quality Management & Business Excellence* 17(1): 117-130.

549   Waldman JD, Arora S, Smith HL, Hood JN. 2006. Improving medical practice outcomes by retaining clinicians. *Journal of Medical Practice Management* March/April pp. 263-271.

550   Waldman JD. 2006. Change the Metrics: If *you get what you measure*, then measure what you want—retention." *Journal of Medical Practice Management* July/August, pp. 1-7.

551   Waldman JD, Hood JN, Smith HL. 2006. Healthcare CEO and Physician—Reaching Common Ground. *J of Healthcare Mgmt.* May/June 51(3): 171-187

552   Waldman JD, Yourstone SA, Smith HL. 2007. Learning-*The* Means to Improve Medical Outcomes. *Health Services Mgmt Research* 2007; 20: 227-237.

553   Waldman JD, Smith HL. 2007. Thinking Systems need Systems Thinking. *Systems Research and Behavioral Science* 24: 1-15.

554   Waldman JD, Cohn K. September 2007. Mend the *Gap*. In The Business of Health, Editors: KH Cohn & D Hough, Praeger Perspectives, New York.

555   Waldman JD. 2009. The Triple Standard in Healthcare. *Calif J Politics & Policy* 1(1): 1-13.

556   Waldman JD. 2010. Uproot U.S. Healthcare. ADM Books: Albuquerque, NM.

557   Waldman JD. 2010. Cambio Radical al Sistema de Salud de los Estados Unidos. ADM Books: Albuquerque, NM

558   Waldman JD. 2013. THE HEALTH OF HEALTHCARE (I): The Right Approach is Medical. *Journal Medical Practice Mgmt*, In Press.

559   Walker J, Pan Eric, Douglas J, Adler-Milstein J, Bates DW, Middleton B. January 2005. The Value of Health Care Information Exchange And Interoperability. *Heath Affairs*. W 5—10-18.

560   *Wall Street Journal* Editorial, January 2, 2003. Lawyers vs. Patients---III, p. A14.

561   *Wall Street Journal Online*. May 10, 2011. "National Health Preview: RomneyCare's bad outcomes keep coming." Accessed at: http://online.wsj.com/article/SB1000142405274870386420457631337052 7615288.html?mod=googlenews_wsj.

562   Wallach EJ. 1983. Individuals and organizations: The cultural match. *Training and Development Journal* 37: 29-36.

563   Walshe K, Rundall TG. 2001. Evidence-based management: From theory to practice in health care." *Millbank Quarterly* 79(3): 429-457

564   Ward CJ. 1991. Analysis of 500 obstetric and gynecologic malpractice claims: Causes and prevention. *Am J Obstet Gynecol* 165: 298306.

565   Watts, AW. 1951. The Wisdom of Insecurity. Pantheon Books: New York.

566   Watson GH. 2002. Peter F. Drucker: Delivering Value to Customers. *Quality Progress* May pp. 55-61.

567   Weber J, Wheelwright S. 1997. Massachusetts General Hospital: CABG Surgery (A). *Harvard Business School Case* # 9-696-015

568   Weick KE. 1993. The collapse of sensemaking in organizations: The Mann Gulch Disaster. *Administrative Science Quarterly* 38: 628-652.

569   Weil TP. 1987. The changing relationship between physicians and the hospital CEO. *Trustee* Feb; 40(2): 15-18.

570   Weil PA. 1990. Job turnover of CEOs in teaching and nonteaching hospitals. *Academic Med* 65(1): 1-7.

571   Weisman CS, Alexander CS, Chase GA. 1981. Determinants of hospital staff nurse turnover. *Medical Care* 19(4): 431-443.

572   Wickline v. State, 192 Cal. App.3d 16.0.1645 (1986), 239 Cal.Rptr. 805,825.

573   Wicks E. 2007. Human Rights and Healthcare. Hart Publishing: Portland, OR.

574   Wiener, Y. 1988. Forms of value systems: A focus on organizational effective-ness, cultural change, and maintenance. *Acad of Mgt Rev* 13: 534-545.

575   Wilcox FK. 1993. Corporate culture in a mythless society. *Amer Journal of Medical Quality* 1993; 8: 134-7.

576   Wilson CN, Meadors AC. 1990. Hospital Chief Executive Officer Turnover. *Hospital Topics* 68(1): 35-39.

577   Wilson CN, Stranahan H. 2000. Organizational characteristics associated with hospital CEO turnover. *Journal of Health Care Management* 45(6): 395-404.

578   Wilson L. July 22, 2004. Healthier habits will reduce medical costs. *Albuquerque Journal* A13.

579   Winton R, March 18, 2009. Former City of Angels hospital executive pleads guilty to paying kickbacks. Accessed March 2009 at: http://latimes.com/news/local/la-me-medfraud19-2009mar19,0,934741.story.

580   Wise LC. 1990. Tracking turnover. *Nursing Economic$* 8(1): 45-51

581   Wittkower ED, Stauble WJ. 1972. Psychiatry and the general practitioner. *Psychiatry Med* 3:287-301.

582   Wood KM, Matthews GE. 1997. Overcoming the physician group-hospital cultural gap. *Healthcare Financial Management* 51:69-70.

583   Woods, TE. 2009. Meltdown. Regenery Publishing: Washington, DC.

584   Woolhandler S, Campbell T, Himmelstein DU. 2003. Costs of Health Care Administration in the United States and Canada. *NEJM* 349:768-775.

585   Wu AW, Cavanaugh TA, McPhee SJ, Lo B, Micco GP. 1997. To tell the truth—Ethical and Practical Issues in disclosing medical mistakes to patients. *J Gen Intern Med* 12: 770-775.

586   Wysocki B. April 9, 2004. To fix health care, hospitals take tips from factory floor. *Wall Street Journal* A6.

587   Yelle LE. 1979. The Learning Curve—Historical Review and Comprehensive Survey. *Decision Sciences* 302–28.

588   Yeung KO, Brockbank JW, Ulrich DO. 1991. Organizational culture and human resource practices: an empirical assessment. *Research in Organizational Change and Development* 5: 59-82.

589   Young GJ, Charns MP, Daley J, et al. Best Practices for Managing Surgical Services: The Role of Coordination. *Health Care Management Review* 1997; 22(4): 72-81.

590   Zammuto RF, Krakower JY. 1991. Quantitative and qualitative studies of organizational culture. *Res in Organizational Change and Development* 5:83-114.

591   Zimmerman R, Oster C. June 24, 2002. Insurers' missteps helped provoke malpractice 'crisis.' *Wall Street Journal*, pp 1, 8.

592   Zuger, A. 2004. Dissatisfaction with Medical Practice. *New England Journal of Medicine* 350(1): 69-76

Glossary of Healthcare Terms

Dr. Deane's glossary of terms and phrases in healthcare is purely functional. It is not an academic dictionary. It is intended to facilitate dialogue about healthcare between ordinary people. To converse successfully, we need to have a common language. Unfortunately, many words, phrases and abbreviations used in healthcare may not mean what you think.

Thus, what I mean when I write the word "cost" may not convey that same meaning to you when you see the word "cost." We must agree on terms before we can communicate successfully. I hope you find this glossary helpful. I know you will find it instructive, sometimes surprising, and even amusing.

➤ **Healthcare** versus **health care**—As one word, healthcare means a huge system that consumes 1/6th of U.S. annual GDP. Health care— two words—refers to a close personal (fiduciary) service relationship, protected by law, between a patient and a provider.

➤ **ACA**—Affordable Care Act also known colloquially as Obamacare. We should use the full name—Patient Protection and Affordable Health Care Act of 2010 (PPAHCA)—to keep in our minds what it was supposed to do for us.

➤ **Adverse impact**—where a patient is harmed during (not necessarily by) health care. This is a negative patient outcome such as failure to improve, or being sicker/worse after treatment. Contrast this *outcome* or result to the words error or mistake (see below) that refer to a *behavior* or action, not an outcome. Read about this important distinction in detail in "Uproot U.S. Healthcare."

➤ **APTC**—Advanced Premium Tax Credit aka "ACA subsidies" refers to the money offered by the federal government to offset the costs of health insurance premiums. There is a sliding scale downward from 100% support at 139% of poverty line and below, to 400% of the poverty line (≈$92,000/year), where subsidies cease. This means that 79% of the U.S. population qualifies for subsidy.

➤ **Big Pharma**— a common acronym for huge, usually multinational pharmaceutical companies, such as GlaxoSmithKline, Johnson & Johnson, Merck, Pfizer, and Roche.

➤ **Bureaucracy**—excessively complicated administrative process or system. For my purposes, "bureaucracy" includes (1) administration such as eligibility, confirmation, billing, coding, payment, and distribution; (2) insurance activities from actuarial analysis to authorization; and (3) the regulatory machine from rule-making through review process to compliance oversight and accreditation/de-accreditation.

➤ **Butterfly effect**—is a crude way of describing the Law of Disproportionate Consequences. This "law" states that small actions can have big outcomes and conversely, grand actions can have trivial or insignificant results.

➤ **Cadillac Tax**—This is part of PPAHCA. It levies a 40% tax on any insurance premium that costs annually more than $10,200 for an individual or $27,500 for a family. This tax has little to do with personal income and everything to do with benefits of the insurance plan. The Cadillac tax will hit those in high-risk occupations such as construction workers, firemen, and police.

➤ **Cancer**—where a previously healthy cell in a human body or part of a system no longer performs its normal functions, and begins to grow uncontrollably, ultimately killing the person or the system.

➤ **CBO**—Congressional Budget Office is tasked with predicting the *future* economic and budgetary effects of Congressional action. For example, the CBO has variously calculated the future cost of

PPAHCA as low as $1.1 trillion and as high as $1.7 trillion. Contrast CBO to GAO (below).

➢ **Charge** (price)—what you see on a Bill for Payment. This has no relationship, repeat no relationship, to what is actually paid or to the cost.

➢ **CLASS Act** (Community Living Assistance Services and Support)—Was Title VII part of PPAHCA. It was intended to create a voluntary, public long-term care insurance program, but was deleted from the Act by the White House seven months after PPAHCA was signed into Law.

➢ **Complexity**—According to the dictionary, complex means "composed of many different and connected parts." It also means "not easy to understand." Complexity in healthcare comes in two forms: inherent and artificial.

➢ **Concierge medicine**—also called direct-pay medicine. This refers to doctors who do not accept insurance but rather have the patients pay them directly. This usually involves a retainer fee that covers office visits. Most direct-pay practices negotiate on behalf of their patients very large discounts at labs and with hospitals as well as pharmacies, because the patients will pay cash. By cutting out the insurance carriers, these practices dramatically reduce both their administrative expenses and the time doctors now spend on bureaucratic nonsense.

➢ **Consumer** (in health care this is the patient)—It is important to recognize that healthcare is a third party payer system, meaning the consumer (of goods and services) is not the payer. She or he does not directly pay the supplier (provider) for the services and goods consumed. Thus, there is micro-economic disconnection (see below), where supply and demand—normally connected supplier competition and demander's money—are *disconnected*. This prevents the functioning of free market forces.

➢ **Cosmology episode**—a condition where the world makes no sense, where for instance, the sun rises out of the south. This is what providers of health care face every day. They think they are doing what patients want and yet the "system" in which they work obstructs, constrains and punishes them. This makes no sense—a cosmology episode.

➤ **Cost**—is the most misunderstood and therefore misused word in healthcare language. You and I use "cost" to mean the sum of all materials, labor, and capital to produce a product or service. Using that definition, no one knows the cost of anything in health care as well as healthcare. In the world of healthcare, "cost" is allocated, apportioned, back calculated, and projected, but not the simple sum of all factors of production and distribution. Be sure you understand that anyone who claims to report the true cost of anything in healthcare is guessing.

➤ **Covered Life**—someone who has signed up with a qualified health plan for insurance. As soon as the insurance card is issued, the person is covered for 90 days, even if that individual does not pay the premiums.

➤ **Defensive medicine**—when providers make decisions based on how their record will look, not necessarily on what is best for the patient.

➤ **Diagnosis**—literally means "the identification of the *nature* of an illness." Nature can mean only the description of the ailment and/ or it can mean the root cause of your problem. Many, in fact most, diagnoses are descriptive, not etiologic (see root cause).

➤ **(To) Dissolve** (a problem)—this is the most desirable of the four ways to "solve" a problem and is described in detail "Uproot U.S. Healthcare." To dissolve a problem means you change the system so the root cause of the problem no longer exists. Therefore, the problem cannot recur because it no longer exists.

➤ **"Donut hole"**—a gap in coverage in Medicare (Part D) where the beneficiary has to pay all of his/her prescription drug costs. The gap is between where the initial/minimum coverage ends, and when the beneficiary has spent enough to reach the catastrophic coverage threshold.

➤ **Effectiveness** (contrast to effectiveness)—refers to how successful a person, organization, or system is in achieving the desired effect. In baseball, an effective pitcher is one who throws strikes that people cannot hit. An effective healthcare system makes and keeps the most people as healthy and as long-lived as possible. *An effective system is always efficient, but an efficient one may not be effective.*

➤ **Efficiency** (contrast to efficiency)—is classically defined in terms of work per unit time, but it really means using the least resources (money, labor, power) while working. You can be very efficient and still be ineffective. If you can produce ten buggy whips per hour but nobody wants to buy them, you are highly efficient but not effective (at producing income for your manufacturing company.) In healthcare, if you see ten patients per hour, you are very efficient. If they all stay sick, you are very ineffective.

➤ **EMTALA**—Emergency Medical Transport and Active Labor Act of 1986, also known as the anti-dumping law. This requires emergency rooms to care (rather than transfer) any acutely, seriously ill patient regardless of whether or not the patient has any payment source. EMTALA created the *unfunded mandate.*

➤ **Entitlement**—a legal right or just claim to receive or do something. Most people use the words right and entitlement interchangeably, assuming they are free (no payment); everyone gets it whenever they want (on their time frame); regardless of income, location, age, and for health care—regardless of citizenship.

➤ **Error/mistake** [contrast to adverse impact]—an incorrect action or behavior. To make an error requires that the correct action or behavior is known and possible. So in healthcare, if there is no medical choice that is proven to be "correct," then there cannot be a mistake, even if a patient has an adverse impact (see above).

➤ **Exemption** (or waiver)—means that some organization does not have to comply with the legal requirements of PAHCA. Certain religious groups and over 1400 organization—unions or businesses—have been granted exemptions.

➤ **FFM**—Federally-Facilitated Marketplace. This is the federally run program, created by PPAHCA, where American citizens can (and must by law) purchase health insurance. The website's URL is www.healthcare.gov.

➤ **Fiduciary**—a relationship between two people where person "A" gives power/control to person "B" to use for the benefit of person "A".

➤ **GAO**—Government Accounting Office. Where the CBO is concerned with the future, the GAO, also called the "Congressional watchdog," looks at the past. This agency assesses the spending that occurred. For instance, in 1990 on the twenty-fifth anniversary of the Medicare Act, the GAO calculated how much was actually spent in contrast to how much was budgeted/predicted in 1965. Congress under-estimated the cost of Medicare by 854%.

➤ **Guaranteed issue**—rule that requires insurance carriers to accept any patient for coverage, regardless of any pre-existing health condition the patient might have and thus regardless of how much that individual might cost the insurance Plan.

➤ **Health Insurance Exchange**—a major component of PPAHCA where people can shop for health insurance and those who qualify (70% of U.S. population) can obtain subsidies to reduce out-of-pocket costs. Eighteen States are operating their own exchanges. The majority has decided not to create State-based Exchanges: their citizens must obtain insurance through the FFM (see above) at www.healthcare.gov.

➤ **"Healthcare is a sick patient."**—This is my way of saying that only a medical approach can fix healthcare. The political and financial attempts over the past fifty years have made patient Healthcare sicker.

➤ **High Risk Pool**—refers to those Americans with expensive, usually chronic medical conditions whose annual medical expenses make it difficult-to-impossible to obtain health insurance.

➤ **HIPAA**—Health Insurance Portability and Accountability Act of 1996. Intended to solve the problem of losing health insurance when losing a job—it did nothing to fix this. HIPAA created a massive regulatory machine, a host of burdensome rules, and tens of billions in costs, all supposedly to protect the confidentiality of medical information (it doesn't).

- ➤ **HITECH** (Health Information Technology for Economic and Clinical Health) Act—was part of The American Recovery and Reinvestment Act of 2009. It was intended to create medical information technology standards and infrastructure and to strengthen the security of personal health information.

- ➤ **Incentive**—is a motivator that either encourages someone to perform some behavior (colloquially called a "carrot" or reward), or to not do something (a "stick" or punishment). Low prices, say for insurance, are a positive incentive to purchase. PPAHCA's tax penalty for not buying insurance is a negative incentive or "stick."

- ➤ **Independent Payment Advisory Board** (IPAB)—created by PPAHCA, this federal agency is tasked with reducing health care spending. It is imperative that you read more about this secretive committee as it will directly impact what care you can receive and what may be denied to you. IPAB was recently renamed HTAC (Health Technology Assessment Committee). IPAB was what former Governor Sarah Palin famously called a "Death Panel" in 2009.

- ➤ **Individual mandate**—refers to the cornerstone of PPAHCA: a federal mandate or requirement that each citizen (does not apply to non-citizens or illegals) purchase health insurance. This was struck down by the Supreme Court, which then said it would be constitutional if it were called a tax.

- ➤ **Insurance principle**—"where small contributions of the many pay the great (large) expenses of the few." Lots of people put small amounts of money into a common "risk pool" and a small number of people take out large amounts of money.

- ➤ **"It just stands to reason."**—A phrase used by those who have no hard evidence to support their position or plan. They rely on appeal to emotion.

- ➤ **"Job lock"**—being stuck in a job you do not want to do because you will lose your insurance benefits if you leave. In February 2014 the CBO released a report predicting that PPAHCA would cause the loss of over two million jobs in the U.S. The previous House Minority leader, Nancy Pelosi, hailed this result saying that Americans would no longer "be joblocked but [as a result of PPAHCA, they would be able] to follow their passion," meaning they could work at what they chose, or not work at all.

> **Learn**—to acquire data, knowledge, understanding and (hopefully) wisdom. To learn requires you to question what you have been taught is true, and sometimes unlearn that so you can learn what IS true. As I have written, "Today's 'best medical practice' can be tomorrow's malpractice."

> **Market failure**—market here mean a "free market," where consumers spend their own money and where prices can vary. Market failure means that the free market does not allocate goods and services *efficiently*, giving the best and cheapest stuff to the most people. The usual alternative suggested to a free market is central (government) control, which has been shown over and over to be *inefficient*—giving more to some people and little-or-nothing to most others. (This is not Deane's conservative bias or leaning. It is based on history and hard evidence.)

> **Medicaid**—This is an *entitlement* program, in contrast to Medicare. You qualify by low income, age, or having certain chronic conditions. You pay nothing and receive benefits dictated by the government.

> **Medical malpractice** (tort) system—When a patient is injured or harmed in relation to medical care, the malpractice system supposedly punishes the wrongdoer and compensates the injured. An alternative system is proposed in this book, called The Office of Medical Injuries (OMIn).

> **Medicare** (contrast to Medicaid)—This is *not* an entitlement program. You paid into it for your whole working life. Medicare was conceived as a giant Health Savings Account, where you put in money for 40 years and when you retire, that very large pot of money, which accumulated and grew, would pay all the medical expenses of your "golden years." Read here how and why Congress subverted Medicare.

➤ **"Metal level"**—Insurance plans that are ACA-compliant have different amounts (percent) of the costs of your health care that are covered by the Plan. These different levels are signified by using the names of metals: Bronze (60% of your costs are covered); Silver (70%); Gold (80%); and Platinum (90%). Of course, the cost of the insurance premium goes up considerably depending on which "metal" level you choose.

➤ **Micro-economic disconnection**—refers to the separation of the consumer from control of his or her own money. This makes it impossible for the free market to function, as supply and demand can no longer balance each other.

➤ **Moral hazard**—refers to the danger (to society) of spending other people's money and therefore having no need to act responsibly or economize.

➤ **Navigator**—PPAHCA requires each State to have people available to help individuals through the complexity of purchasing health insurance. These individuals are presumably impartial (not paid by or beholden to any insurance carrier, as brokers can be). Navigators can also be called "in-person assisters."

➤ **Net** (when calculating pretty much anything)—I frequently use this word because too many people look exclusively at the short term cost, without considering long term costs and without evaluating benefits at all. A "net calculation" for spending on healthcare would determine **value**—what we *really* care about—by comparing long-term costs and risks to long-term benefits to patients.

➤ **Payer**—can be confusing. In most aspects of your life, the payer IS the **consumer**, they are one and the same. In a free market, the consumer/payer gives money to the supplier in exchange for goods and services. Healthcare, with its third party payer system, is not a free market. The consumer does not directly pay the supplier and therefore is not the payer. The **supplier** (provider) does not set his/her price. The government, not the market, determines the price. There is a third party **payer** who either has no incentive to economize (the government) or is rewarded (incentivized) when it denies payment for care (insurance).

➤ **PCIP** (Pre-Existing Condition Insurance Program)—A component of ACA that was supposed to provide insurance for those usually *uninsurable* because of [expensive] pre-existing medical conditions. Enrollment was discontinued with less than a third of the eligible people signed up. The Chairman of the New Mexico High Risk Insurance Pool said, "Washington just left the sickest of Americans high and dry, holding nothing but an empty promise."

➤ **Perverse incentive**—means that someone is rewarded when they do the opposite of what is wanted. In retail, this would be giving a bonus to the person who sells the least products. In healthcare, it is perverse when insurance makes profit by delaying, deferring, or denying medical care —the three D's in chapter 2— even though you need it, now!

➤ *Primum non nocere*—Latin phrase considered the "prime directive" for physicians. Typically MIS-translated as "First (above all), do no harm." However, a more precise interpretation of the Latin yields, "<u>At least</u>, do no harm!"

➤ **Provider** (of health care)—anyone whose activities *directly* affect a patient, such as a doctor, nurse, respiratory therapist, social worker, etc. Many others, not called providers, *indirectly* affect patient welfare, such as billers, coders, managers, legislators, regulators, support staff, technicians, etc.

➤ **Psychic reward**—an emotional or psychological, non-material payment for a service, product, or action. For most health care providers, the psychic reward for helping others is more important than the monetary.

➤ **"Public option"**—is a short-hand colloquial term for single payer, in contrast to having multiple entities, usually insurance carriers but sometimes health organizations, who pay the costs for health care goods and services. Many use the Canadian system as an example of a public option. See "single payer."

➢ **Rescission**—insurance industry jargon for cancelling an insurance policy, often for frivolous reasons or with a trumped up excuse.

➢ **Right** (to health care)—means you are entitled to health care (the service), when you want, where you want, what you want, for free, without needing to qualify in any way. Proponents say that by simply being alive, you have this right. The relationship between a right to health care and one's personal responsibility has never been openly discussed. I believe the lack of consensus on this matter is at the heart of problems in our healthcare system.

➢ **Root cause** (etiology is the medical term)—refers to the primary or first cause. This is the "why" of illness. In diabetes, the symptoms are related to elevated sugar in the blood, but elevated sugar is not the root cause, which is due to failure of insulin to regulate blood sugar. Dysfunction or improper production of insulin is the root cause in diabetes. Has anyone shown to you what the root causes are to explain why our healthcare system is "broken"?

➢ **"Romneycare"**—colloquial term for the Massachusetts health care insurance reform Act signed into law while Mitt Romney was Governor (April 2006). The proper name for this system is Commonwealth Care.

➢ **SCOTUS**—common abbreviation for Supreme Court of the United States

➢ **SHOP**—abbreviation for the Small Business Health Options Program, which is part of the ACA.

➢ **Signup** (Enrollee)—Washington counts anyone who has completed the application process for insurance, even if that person is not covered (no card issued) and/or has never paid premiums.

➢ **Single payer system**—where the government is the distribution source for payments to providers, institutions, suppliers, and (if insurance is used), insurance middlemen. Since it controls the money, the government dictates how much it will pay and what it will pay for. There are no market forces in a single payer system as there is no free market: a monopoly (government) controls both supply and demand. The U.S. Veterans Administration is a single payer system, as is the British National Health Service. See "public option."

> **Spending** (noun)—money paid. All too often, spending is mistakenly used as the same as cost, which (see above) is very different.

> **Subsidy** from ACA—see: **APTC.**

> **System** (contrast to process)—a set of connected things or parts that form a complex structure. The key is the word connected, without the structure and connections, it is just a pile of things or parts and can do nothing.

> **Systems thinking**—a management approach that emphasizes the need to study the intact system or entire structure as a whole. When you break it up and study each part separately, you lose the connections and it's "system-ness." Practicing good medicine (on anything) requires systems thinking. A good doctor would never do something to improve kidney function without considering how that treatment might affect the heart, lungs, or liver.

> **TANSTAAFL**—"There ain't no such thing as a free lunch." It means that nothing in this world is free, nothing. *Someone* has to pay for it, whatever "it" is.

> **The Three D's**—a strategy used by health care payers to hold on to your money as long as possible: delay, defer, or deny.

> **Two-master dilemma**—the problem of who should be your first priority: your employer or your customer; your patient's best interests or following regulations. I call this the "who-master dilemma."

> **"Trust me! I have your best interests at heart."**—A common catchphrase of those who take a paternalistic attitude toward others and control them.

> **UMRA**—Unfunded Mandate Reform Act of 1995. This Act was intended to fix the problem created by EMTALA (see above) which created the unfunded mandate: the law that requires hospitals to treat patients for free, which in turn makes them overcharge paying

patients to avoid bankruptcy. As you can see, UMRA did not resolve the unfunded mandate, which is an even bigger problem in 2014 than it was in 1995.

- ➢ **Uncompensated care**—medical care that a hospital must provide (by law) for which it receives no payment—the unfunded mandate. This was an unintended consequence EMTALA (see above).

- ➢ **Underinsured**—The purpose of insurance is to prevent financial disaster in the event of an expensive medical catastrophe. As many as 84 million Americans who have medical insurance may not have enough coverage to protect them from medical bankruptcy. These are the "<u>under</u>insured."

- ➢ **Uninsured**—those who have no medical insurance. Current estimates put this number at 45-50 million Americans, 24% of whom are not legal citizens.

- ➢ **Universal health care**—national healthcare systems where reputedly everyone gets care. I write "reputedly" because these systems are not *universal* (non-citizens do not get free care); *care may be denied* by government decree; and often (viz., Canada), you cannot get care when you need it.

- ➢ **"We The Patients"**—is how I refer to We The People (all Americans) while emphasizing that every individual is now a patient or eventually will be a patient. We The Patients includes Democrats and Republicans; rich and poor; all ages and stages; and citizens as well as Americans here illegally. If you are alive in the U.S., you are part of We The Patients. We are all in this together. By "this" I mean life.

Fixing Our Medical Malpractice Problem

In chapter 3, I promised a solution for a U.S. medical malpractice (med-mal) system that doesn't do what We The Patients want from it. It fails because it was based on the adversarial, tort law system. If the root cause is the design model, the answer is to replace it with a different model. *Reforming* the current system will not get us what we want. We need to *replace* it. THAT is the **OMIn** (Office of Medical Injuries)a replacement for the current tort-based system.

The OMIn will give us what the public wants: (1) Help those who are injured during health care; and (2) Provide for and encourage learning so we can have better outcomes tomorrow than are possible today.

OMIn will require enabling legislation, including creation of a secure national medical database. The current med-mal system will not be officially dismantled but injured patients will be offered *either* the current tort system *or* the OMIn, not both.

OMIn will have four Divisions: Compensation; Dissolution; Improvements; and Oversight. Financing is surprisingly straightforward.

Compensation Division

Any medical injury can be reported by the injured patient, a family member, or an involved medical professional. The Compensation Section, staffed with medical experts and actuaries, will evaluate the facts of the injury, determine the severity and time of dysfunction related to the injury and offer appropriate compensation. The Compensation Division can request additional medical information, even tests, in order to make its determinations. This Division will also accept testimonial and other evidence submitted by the family or patient.

The patient can, at his or her choosing, offer a different calculation for compensation based on advice from experts retained by the injured party at his/her expense. The Compensation Division will review the additional data and analysis. If it deems necessary, the Division will amend the proposed compensation scheme.

Within 90 days of completion of its analysis, the Compensation Division will pass the case file with all the facts on to both the Dissolution and Oversight Divisions (see below).

Dissolution Division

To "dissolve" a problem means to change the system so that the problem ceases to exist and therefore can never recur. The Dissolution Division is tasked with learning from the experience involved in the injury. The Division will work in concert with the involved local professionals and the Healthcare Institution where the injury occurred to determine how and why the injury occurred and if possible, to design a way to prevent the injury from ever happening again.

The Dissolution Division will be staffed with consulting experts in both medical and management areas, from subspecialties such as Cardiology and Endocrinology to Operations, Organizational Behavior, and Technologic Innovation.

Sometimes the cause of an injury cannot be determined. In such cases, a dissolving recommendation may not be possible. In most cases, a way can be devised to prevent recurrence. The Dissolution Division will not only help develop such an improvement but monitor the implementation of the change in the Institution or system where the injury occurred.

The Dissolution Division is required to pass on its findings to the Improvement Division within 90 days of completion of study and design of change. It is not required to wait until the change has been implemented and tested.

Improvements Division

The Improvements Division will be staffed in a similar manner to the Dissolution Division with consultants in both medical and management areas, from subspecialties such as Cardiology and Endocrinology to Operations, Organizational Behavior, and Technologic Innovation.

The Improvements Division receives all the findings and specific recommendations from the Dissolution Division. It collates and analyzes this data looking for trends and for improvements that can be generalized: Improvements that would work in many facilities rather than just the one where the original injury occurred. When such improvements are found, they are distributed to all U.S. healthcare facilities by online distribution as well as to the Oversight Division. The Improvements Division is not tasked with overseeing the implementation of such recommended improvements. It is required only to distribute the information. Implementation is left to the discretion of each healthcare system or institution.

Oversight Division

All case files as well as all recommended improvements are shared with the Oversight Division, which looks for patterns of recurring medical injuries after the wide distribution of a Dissolution Recommendation specific to that injury. Either the recommendation does not work (and the injuries recur) or institutions are being negligent. The Division, staffed primarily with experts in medicine, is tasked with determining trends and differentiating (A) recommendation failure from (B) institution failure. When the Division decides it is (A), the Oversight Division confers with the Improvements Division to modify the Recommendation and then distribute the revision. When the determination is (B), the case is referred to appropriate disciplinary services, be it medical society, professional organization or an accreditation body such as The Joint Commission, formerly the Joint Commission on Accreditation of Healthcare Organizations.

Financing the OMIn

As everyone benefits from the OMIn, everyone should pay for the OMIn. Like Social Security, there will be a large time lag between a person's payment into the OMIn and the need for compensation to an individual injured patient. Of course, it is hoped that like all catastrophic insurance, the individual will never need the OMIn, but we know many will.

It is presently impossible to predict accurately how much the OMIn will cost but a reasonable upper limit would be $20 billion per year. This is less than any current estimate of the cost of defensive medicine alone and a small fraction of the current cost of medical liability insurance as well as legal costs, all of which will disappear as the OMIn replaces the med-mal system. Net savings to the nation will exceed $100 billion per year.

A new tax will be added to what is now the Social Security tax, called OMIn tax. This money will be sequestered from the General Fund and accounted separately so that the actual expenses of OMIn can be easily determined. The OMIn tax will be adjusted, most likely downward, in subsequent years.

Index

U, V, W, X, Y, Z

CPSIA information can be obtained
at www.ICGtesting.com
Printed in the USA
FSOW01n1705111215
14078FS